HEARING AIDS FROM THE INSIDE OUT

HEARING AIDS FROM THE INSIDE OUT

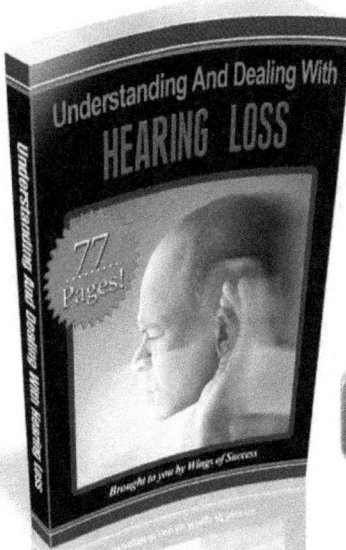
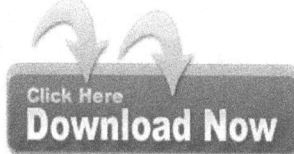
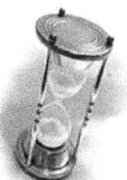

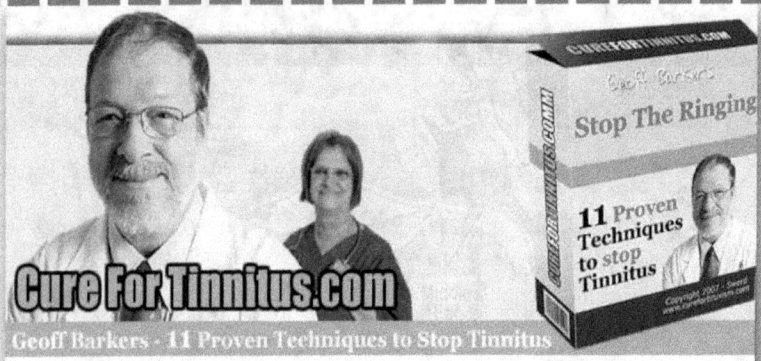

At Last! A complete program to eliminate that annoying ringing noise in your ears and end Tinnitus for good!

I have put every Tinnitus remedy to the test and now the results are in...

"Finally, you find out the real way to end Tinnitus for good. His step-by-step program reveals how to seriously reduce or even cure Tinnitus in just a few minutes a day!"

- What exactly is Tinnitus? (There are some things about your condition that I guarantee you don't know yet. Get the hard facts at page 3)
- The best treatment for YOU (Get a personalized treatment on page 8)
- The fastest way to STOP the ringing noise (discover this at page 9)
- Get the 6 secret recipes that can stop YOUR Tinnitus (Look at this breakthrough on page 15)
- Prevent Tinnitus the easy way (I bet you didn't consider this every time you went to work! Live by the rules on page 17)
- Proven remedies that can work for you. Choose from 11 Tinnitus remedies that you can perform yourself, right now in the office or at home. (Get hold of this priceless information on pages 18 - 24!)

DOWNLOAD NOW

"Sensational Breakthrough Movement Exposes The Revolutionary Ways To Attract And Manifest Anything You Want In Life, Like Magic!"

Long-Kept Secrets Never Before Explained About How To Create The Life Of Your Dreams Finally Revealed In Startling Materials!

DOWNLOAD NOW

HARNESS THE HIDDEN LAWS OF THE UNIVERSE

HEARING AIDS FROM THE INSIDE OUT

Contents

An Introduction To Hearing Aids..................9
History Of Hearing Aids..................10
Hearing Loss And Hearing Aids..................12
Types Of Hearing Aids..................13
Before You Get Hearing Aids..................14
Maintaining Your Hearing Aids..................15
Hearing Aids And Children..................16
Batteries For Hearing Aids..................17
Hearing Aids: Policies And Warranties..................18
Hearing Aids: Just One Or Two?..................19
Hearing Aids Pain..................21
All About Open Fit Hearing Aids..................22
Are Deals On BTE Hearing Aids By Mail Too Good To Be True?..................24
Have You Heard Of Beltone Hearing Aids?..................26
How Phonak Hearing Aids Make Listening Easy..................28
Siemens Artis Hearing Aids May Be The Solution For You..................30
The Benefits Of Starkey Hearing Aids..................32
What To Look For In Inexpensive Hearing Aids..................34
What You Need To Know About To Compare Hearing Aids..................36
What You Should Know About Digital Hearing Aids..................38
Would You Take A Chance On A Cheap Hearing Aid?..................40
Finding The Right Digital Hearing Aids For You..................42
Knowing If Your Child Needs Hearing Aids..................43
Digital Hearing Aids And Other Types..................44
Differences Between Digital Hearing Aids And Others..................46
Knowing When It's Time For Hearing Aids..................48
Do You Have The Proper Hearing Aids?..................50
Digital Hearing Aids For Older Parents..................51
Pros And Cons Of Digital Hearing Aids..................52
Basic Knowledge Of Digital Hearing Aids..................53
Digital Hearing Aids Versus Analog..................55
Telecoil Hearing Aids..................56

Hearing Aids Inside Out

Do You Need Hearing Aids? 62
Shopping For Hearing Aids 63
Maintaining Your Hearing Aids 65
Improvements To Hearing Aids 67
Disposable Hearing Aids 68
BTE Hearing Aids Deals 71
The Importance Of Hearing Aids 73
What Does Siemens Have To Offer? 75
Where To Find Discount Digital Hearing Aids 77
The Popularity Of Behind The Ear Hearing Aids 79
Siemens Artis Hearing Aids And Their Popularity 81
Why Use Hearing Aids For Dogs? 83
BTE Digital Hearing Aids 85
Choosing Discount Hearing Aids 87
Good Things To Know About Siemens Hearing Aids 89
Hearing Aids GA: For A Good Fit 91
How Do Hearing Aids Work? 93
How Low Cost Hearing Aids Can Change Your Life 95
The Variety Of Oticon Hearing Aids 97
Choices In BTE Hearing Aids 99
The Importance Of Getting The Best Hearing Aid 101
Beltone Hearing Aids 103
Phonak Hearing Aids 105
Siemens Artis Hearing Aids May Be The Solution For You 107
Starkey Hearing Aids 109

An Introduction To Hearing Aids

It is estimated that more than 28 million people in the US have a significant loss of hearing. For the majority of these people, a hearing aid will probably be the best way to improve their hearing. Recent advancements in hearing aid technology mean that modern hearing aids have a high level of sound quality in a very small device. It should be noted that a hearing aid will not restore normal hearing. What it can do is make it easier for the user to detect and interpret sounds. Often someone who is hard of hearing will not notice if someone is trying to speak to them. This is what a hearing aid will help with.

Although there are several distinct types of hearing aids on the market today, they all work in a similar fashion. A microphone or receiver picks up sound waves and converts them to an electric signal. This signal is then processed and sent to a speaker, which converts it back to an audio signal. The processing serves to amplify those frequencies of which the user has trouble hearing. Hearing aids are able to allow their user to hear human speech at a comfortable volume. This may require some time to adjust to the new signals the brain receives.

Hearing aids are not a perfect solution – they do have their limitations. They will not restore normal hearing, nor will they eliminate background noise. However, they may be adjusted to lessen background noise. New users to hearing aids often complain that their voices sound funny to themselves, and that they are bothered by the relative loud noise from things like refrigerator fans and traffic on the street outside. However, as they have a chance to adapt to their new hearing aid, their brain begins to filter out background noises to a more comfortable level.

There are different types of hearing loss. The two main types are conductive hearing loss and sensorineural hearing loss. Conductive hearing loss occurs when sound waves cannot reach the inner ear. This can be caused by such things as a buildup of earwax, infection, fluid in the ear, or a punctured eardrum. Sensorineural hearing loss occurs when there is damage to the auditory nerve or hair cells in the inner ear. This damage can be the result of loud noise, injury, infection, a genetic condition or aging. While conductive hearing loss can often be corrected by surgery, sensorineural hearing loss can not.

History Of Hearing Aids

A hearing aid is a device that helps someone who has trouble hearing. Hearing aids today are electronic instruments that receive and amplify sounds. The first hearing aids are now known as body worn aids. They are bulky instruments about the size of a deck of cards that are designed to be carried in a pocket. A wire connects the hearing aid to an earphone. Body worn aids are seldom used anymore, except occasionally in the case of very severe hearing loss.

The most common hearing aid type today is the behind the ear aid, or BTE. A behind the ear hearing aid consists of a case that clips behind the ear and is connected directly by plastic sound tubes to a custom molded earpiece. BTE's are used for a wide range of hearing losses. Behind the ear hearing aids generally have a larger battery than other types of hearing aids, allowing them to be more powerful and have a longer life.

With improved technology and miniaturization of electronics, the next generation of hearing aids, in the ear or ITE, became possible. These aids fit in the outer ear bowl. ITE's can be visible to the casual observer. They are also the largest of the custom made styles, and are often the most comfortable, cheapest and simplest to use. Smaller that the in the ear hearing aid is the in the canal, or ITC hearing aid. These aids are usually more expensive than ITE's, and are also harder to adjust owing to the small size of the volume wheel. Going even smaller we find the mini canal, or MC hearing aid. These are the smallest hearing aid you can get that still have a volume adjustment wheel.

The tiniest hearing aids made are the completely in the canal, or CIC hearing aids. They fit so deeply into the ear that they require a removal string. CIC's do not usually have manual controls simply because of their size.

Combining some of the attributes of the behind the ear and the completely in the canal hearing aids are the post auricular canal devices. This design physically separates the processor from the earpiece. The small processor fits behind the ear, while the receiver and speaker portion is imbedded in the earpiece which is placed deep in the ear canal.

Choosing a type of hearing aid is usually making a trade-off between size, price and flexibility.

Hearing Aids Inside Out

The largest hearing aids used today, the BTE's, are generally the cheapest, most powerful, easiest to adjust and the most durable. However, they are also the most conspicuous. BTE's tend to be the best choice for children, however, owing to their durability and the ability to replace the earpiece as the child grows. Other types of hearing aids would have to be replaced periodically when the child outgrows them.

Hearing Loss And Hearing Aids

It is estimated that more than 28 million Americans are hard of hearing. For most, a hearing aid is the appropriate solution. A hearing aid is a device that helps someone who has trouble hearing. Hearing aids today are electronic instruments that receive and amplify sounds. The earliest hearing aids were usually cone-shaped devices that funneled sound towards the ear in order to amplify it. All hearing aids consist of a microphone or receiver to pick up sound waves and convert them to an electric signal. This signal is then processed and sent to a speaker, which converts it back to an audio signal. The processing serves to amplify those frequencies of which the user has trouble hearing.

There two types of hearing loss are conductive hearing loss and sensorineural hearing loss. Conductive hearing loss occurs when sound waves cannot reach the inner ear and are caused by something like a buildup of earwax, infection, fluid in the ear, or a punctured eardrum. Sensorineural hearing loss occurs when there is damage to the auditory nerve or hair cells in the inner ear. Conductive hearing loss is usually corrected by surgery. Sensorineural hearing loss is usually corrected with a hearing aid.

Hearing aids are not a perfect solution – they do have their limitations. They will not restore normal hearing, nor will they eliminate background noise. However, they may be adjusted to lessen background noise. New users to hearing aids often complain that their voices sound funny to themselves, and that they are bothered by the relative loud noise from things like refrigerator fans and traffic on the street outside. However, as they have a chance to adapt to their new hearing aid, their brain begins to filter out background noises to a more comfortable level.

Types Of Hearing Aids

Old style hearing aids are now known as body worn aids. They were relatively large devices about the size of a deck of cards. Body worn aids are seldom used anymore, except occasionally in the case of very severe hearing loss. The most common hearing aid type today is the behind the ear aid, or BTE. A behind the ear hearing aid consists of a case that clips behind the ear and is connected directly by plastic sound tubes to a custom molded earpiece. BTE's are generally more suitable for children, as they are more durable and easier to adapt as the child grows. The next type of hearing aid is the in the ear or ITE hearing aid. These aids fit in the outer ear bowl and can be visible. They are the most comfortable, least expensive, and easiest to use of the custom fitted hearing aids. Smaller that the in the ear hearing aid is the in the canal, or ITC hearing aid. These aids are usually more expensive than ITE's, and are also harder to adjust owing to the small size of the volume wheel. Even smaller than the ITC's are the mini canal, or MC, hearing aid. These are the smallest hearing aid you can get that still have a volume adjustment wheel. The tiniest hearing aids made are the completely in the canal, or CIC hearing aids. They fit so deeply into the ear that they require a removal string. CIC's do not usually have manual controls simply because of their size.

A feature available on many hearing aids is the telecoil. Telecoils allow the hearing aid to pick up magnetic signals and process them as audio signal. Telecoils were originally developed to help those with hearing aids use the telephone. Older telephone produced fairly strong magnetic fields in their earpieces, which could be picked up by the telecoil. Modern phones do not normally produce strong enough magnetic fields, but many phones and other devices are equipped to transmit to a telecoil anyway. Most users find that the telecoil provides better sound quality and allow the user to more easily concentrate on the desired sound, despite any background noise.

Before You Get Hearing Aids

The first step in getting a hearing aid is to visit an ear care professional to get a full hearing test. The professional will measure several different facets of your hearing, including how well you can hear different tones or frequencies, and how well you can discern speech with various levels of background noise. You should discuss with your doctor or audiologist whether a hearing aid is the best solution for you, or whether it is possible to correct your hearing loss through surgery. Next you'll want to investigate the different styles of hearing aids, and select the one that is right for you, your hearing loss, and your lifestyle. Most hearing aid companies offer a trial period, so don't hesitate to try more than one aid. You will want to check out what features are available with the different hearing aids. Two features which are especially useful are telecoil and direct audio input. These allow you to use assistive listening devices which can be purchased for your home and are available at some public locations.

An important consideration is the full cost of the hearing aid, including batteries and repairs. Make sure you ask what the warranty covers, as well as what is the length of the warranty. A person obtaining a hearing aid for the first time will need to take the time to become familiar with their hearing aid. It may be uncomfortable to start, or your voice may sound funny to yourself. Know how to adjust your hearing aid properly, and be sure to return to your audiologist or hearing aid dispenser for a proper adjustment if it is not comfortable.

Maintaining Your Hearing Aids

It is very important to maintain your hearing aid properly. Hearing aids are delicate instruments, and looking after them is vital. You will need to know how to clean your hearing aid by removing wax buildup, how to replace and dispose of batteries and how to remove moisture from the aid. In order to properly maintain your hearing aid you will want a battery tester and spare batteries, silica gel packs and a plastic stethoscope. You will want to keep your hearing aid clean by wiping it daily with a dry tissue. Moisture is the enemy of your hearing aid, so do not wash it, even with a damp cloth. The silica gel packs are used to prevent moisture from getting into your hearing aid while you are not wearing it. The most common maintenance you will have to do is to replace dead batteries. You will want to replace dead batteries immediately. Remember, in order to prolong the battery life you will want turn off your hearing aids when you're not using them.

A plastic stethoscope is a great tool to make sure your hearing aid is functioning correctly. Use the stethoscope to listen to the output of the hearing aid while you adjust it. You will want to test your hearing aid's response to different volumes and sounds and to check for the presence of static and that the hearing aid is not cutting in and out.

The only part of a hearing aid that should be washed is the ear mold piece of a behind the ear hearing aid. You can gently wash it with a mild detergent. A forced air blower can be used to dry the ear mold more quickly.

If you are having any problems with your hearing aid, take it back to the dispenser or audiologist. A badly functioning hearing aid will cause you discomfort, and decrease the benefit you could have received from it.

Hearing Aids And Children

As a child grows, the ear grows as well. The behind the ear style of hearing aid is preferred for children because the ear mold can be replaced separately from the rest of the unit. In the ear hearing aids would have to be replaced completely as the child outgrew them. In addition, behind the ear hearing aids are better for children because the ear mold and hearing aid can be more easily cleaned and maintained, the controls are more easily adjusted and monitored by parents. And as any parent knows, because behind the ear hearing aids are larger and less likely to get lost, this will save you considerable expense in replacements.

For most children, the real need for a hearing aid comes at school. Without being able to hear properly, a child will miss instructions from their teacher, leading to frustration and poor performance. For children with hearing problems, many schools now will provide assistive learning systems. In these systems, the teacher is typically given a microphone, and the signal is sent directly to the hearing impaired student via either a telecoil or direct audio input. This type of set-up tends to be more effective for the child as it eliminates the amplification of background noise.

In the ear hearing aids are not suitable for young children because the aid must then be replaced frequently as the child grows. Once the child is in their teens, however, their ears will have reached their adult size, and they would be able to wear an in the ear hearing aid if so desired.

Batteries For Hearing Aids

You have hearing aids but have a hard time changing the batteries or are not sure when the batteries should be changed. If you are sure that you're hearing aids are on and you aren't hearing right this might not mean that your hearing aids are broke just that it is time to replace the batteries.

For a guideline to help you remember when you should change the batteries in you're hearing aid; you should at least change them every two weeks. Though you might find that this is too often, mark two weeks on a calendar and see when your hearing starts to decrees. You can mark this on the calendar and go by that.

Though your hearing aid batteries might drain faster the longer you leave you're hearing aids on. Make sure that you turn them off during the night; this will save the battery life. Though, if you are using them a lot during the time that you are using them, the batteries will drain faster.

If you have or are going to get digital hearing aid some of these hearing aids have a low battery warning. These hearing aids will beep to tell you that you have so many hours before the battery stop working. This is a great way to remind yourself if you don't remember when you placed in your last set of batteries.

One important thing is to do is to use a good brand of batteries right from the package. There are special batteries cases that you can buy that will help you change the batteries in you're hearing aids. These might be a little but more money but they'll save you time from changing around the small batteries. Once you have changed the batteries a few times, you should have it down pat.

Hearing Aids: Policies And Warranties

With digital hearing aids the technology that are used for these are the best that has been made. You should look at all the researches you need that can help you narrow down what kind of hearing aid that you need. With so many brands that you can pick from you might have a hard time deciding from what you need.

It might be best to start with the top brands. Research what they have to offer. Keep notes of all the information that you find. This will help you remind yourself what you have found and prices. You might even want to look at the companies return policies and see if they have a no risk evaluation period.

If you find a company that has good policies then you should be able to try hearing aids for so many days risk free. This can help you decide if you can use them. Remember that hearing aids are something that will take a while to get use to. You might have to change the volume and make sure that they work for you before you decide to return them.

You might even find that some companies have warranties that you can get. This will be a good idea to buy. Some warranties might only last for a year. But if you look around you might find that there are longer warranties. This is something that will be a plus for you in case something happens to your hearing aids.

There is also a chance that you might get a supply of batteries with the purchase of your hearing aids. This can be a plus, you won't have to go out and look for batteries when they are needed. One thing to make sure that you look for is that you find a company that has offers that can help you.

Hearing Aids: Just One Or Two?

If you've been looking into getting hearing aids and believe that using only one hearing aid will be enough. The answer is no. You have two ears so you need both hearing aids to be on and working for you to be hearing right. Each ear will pick up different sounds for you to process.

If you have been to a doctor and know that you have different hearing in each ear then you should know if you need a different volume for each ear. This is simply done with getting digital hearing aids. These hearing aids can be tuned to the volume you need.

If you are just using one hearing at the moment you might be start realizing that you are missing parts of a conversation. Or maybe you aren't catching words that are spoken to the ear that has no hearing aid. If you know that this is the case then you should get your hearing checked.

Getting your hearing checked can be the quickest way to know if what kind of hearing aids you need. Once you've had your hearing checked and find out that your hearing had decreased. Then you should look into getting digital hearing. These hearing aids will be able to be changed with your hearing needs.

If you know you are planning on getting new hearing aids, with the internet these days you can find hearing aids for sale. This might be a cheaper way to buy your hearing aids then buying them from a local store. If you don't have access to a computer, ask a family member.

Using one hearing aid will not improve your hearing needs. You should be using two hearing aids at all time. It will make your hearing much better and you'll be able to follow conversation and listen to music and TV much easily.

One thing you should at least know some about when you go out to buy anything, more so when you're planning on buying some hearing aids. Knowing terms will help you know what you're looking at when you decide to buy hearing aids. Even if you're a planning on buying digital hearing aids some of the terms below will help you. Some terms you should look for are:

- **Analog**: this type is found the most in hearing aids. They do how ever make all sounds the

same equal in volume.
- **AssistanceListeningDevices**:theseareavarietyofinstruments,(phones,clocks,bbaby monitors, etc) which help the hearing impaired.
- **BehindtheEar**:thesehearingaidsarewornbehindtheears.
- **Cochlear**:apartoftheinnerear.
- **CompletelyintheCanal**:Thishearingaidfitsdownintothecanaloftheearandyouwon't be able to see it. Because of how small this hearing aid is it might not be the right choice for people with severe hearing loss.
- **ConductiveHearingLoss:**hearingimpairmentcausedbyinterferencewithsound.This kind of hearing loss can mean disease, infection or trauma.
- **Decibels**:aunitmeasurementthatrelatestosound.
- **IntheCanal**:ThesearesimilartoCICbutthistypeislargeranddoesn'tfitrightintotheear canal.
- **IntheEar**: Thesehearingaidsaretheykindthatfitintheouterear.Theyareusedfora wide range of hearing loss. This type of hearing aid is larger then others. ITE hearing aids can be used around technology also.

All these terms can help you when you buy your hearing aids. From digital hearing aids to a different type of hearing aid, reaching and knowing what is out there will save you time in finding the right hearing aids.

Hearing Aids Pain

If you have just bought hearing aids and they are causing pain, or even causing other problems you should stop wearing them for a few days and see if the problems go away. If not you should go see a doctor right away. If the pain doesn't go away after not wearing the aids for a few days then you could talk to the maker of you're hearing aids.

There is a chance that your hearing aids are too large for your ears. If that is the problem then you might need to get smaller hearing aids. If they aren't too large, then there is a possibility they have some rough spots on the earring aids that need to be filed down. You will want to take your hearing aids to a specialized to do this.

If you are just buying any kind of digital hearing aids then you should make sure the company you are buying them at, online or not has a so many risk free trial. This will let you know if the hearing aids that you bought will work for you. To do this you need to wear the hearing aids. If you develop pain after so long then you should contact the company and see what they suggest.

You're goal is not to go without you're hearing aids to cut down on the pain. But to stop the pain so you can continue to use you're hearing aids. Trying to let you're ears heal for a while before you wear you're hearing aids.

If you've tried everything, the next best coarse of action is to go to you're doctor. From there you can get you're hearing aids fixed. Make sure that you do get you're hearing aids fixed. You bought you're hearing aids to hear well. They can't help you if you aren't wearing them.

All About Open Fit Hearing Aids

With so many hearing aids on the market to choose from, you may be overwhelmed by the choices offered. In this article, we will discuss open fit hearing aids. With an open fit aid, you don't have to wait for your ear mold to be made and returned to you; so it takes less time to get the product you'll need. Buying these from a dealer is quicker than waiting on a manufacturer. They'll be maintained wherever you choose to purchase yours. Since open fit aids have evolved into more discreet, less bulky aids, made with better colors and user friendly designs of better quality, people are more willing to wear their hearing aids.

It is hard for some people to admit that they need help to function properly physically. Although there is nothing shameful about getting help for your hearing, it is often a matter of pride for a person to be afraid to give in and accept the use of an aid. Children especially have a fear of enduring teasing and insults from other children if they have anything outstandingly different about their appearance. For older adults, it may be interpreted as a sign of weakness or of getting older.

Open fit hearing aids are also known as over-the-ear, or OTE hearing aids. They are made small for the discretion of the wearer, fitting behind the ear with a clear, thin, almost invisible plastic tube going into the ear towards the ear canal.

These aids are actually best for high frequency hearing defects. If you didn't know already, there are many differences from one person to another when it comes to hearing loss. The loss can occur on many different levels and be at different stages. With the open fit aids, you get power and the most circuit options from many other aids for the high frequency defects.

These OTE aids are also called BTE, or behind-the-ear aids. Their plastic tubing and ear mold will conduct the sound and keep the ear mold more open. Children are often best benefited by these open fit aids, although many adults wear them as well. These aids are made with bright colors and decorations for the children.

One of the possible problems a person could have with an open fit hearing aid is if a tiny hairline crack develops in the plastic tubing. You'll want to take great care with your new aid to protect it from abuse, both by yourself or by others. It should never be left where a child could grab it and chew on it or step on it or where any pets could get to it.

Although it is possible to buy hearing aids yourself without being tested, it is always wiser to have an accurate hearing test done to make sure whether or not your hearing condition requires more than just a simple, over-the-counter type hearing aid. Because the ear is such a complex part of the human body, a trained professional is best to get you the preferred help for your condition. Please take your ears seriously!

Are Deals On BTE Hearing Aids By Mail Too Good To Be True?

BTE hearing aids can be very costly if you go to your hearing professional to get them. Some people with hearing loss enjoy the privacy and convenience of ordering BTE hearing aids by mail. They feel that they can get a better deal and save themselves a trip to the doctor's office. But, are these deals too good to be true?

One thing to be aware of is that so-called hearing aids that do not meet FDA guidelines and simply amplify sound are actually known as listening devices. They are very cheap, both in price and in quality. Some BTE hearing aids by mail like this cost as little as $6.99 per ear. In this case, you probably get what you pay for.

If sellers are not going through an ENT doctor, they will be required by the FDA to make sure that you sign a waiver and turn it in to them. They want to make sure that burden rests squarely on your shoulders. And, maybe it should. You do want to make your own decisions about BTE hearing aids by mail, and this is what you will have to do if you choose not to be fitted by an ENT.

In any case, most hearing aid sellers require the results of a hearing test, which can be done by an audiologist. They will not sell the BTE hearing aid by mail without one. An audiologist is simply a person who does tests on hearing They are not medical doctors and cannot determine if you have an illness or other medical condition. However, they can deliver an audiogram that can be used to adjust the settings on a hearing aid.

The best deals on BTE hearing aids by mail, according to price, are to be found on E-Bay. One reconditioned hearing aid was recently sold there for under $70. It was a Beltone brand hearing aid that was said to have cost over $1000 new. The Siemens High Power 278 BTE aid was sold for around $200. Siemens is a well respected brand name as well. Also available by signing a waiver was the Siemens Infinity Pro, which was priced at about $400. If you can't afford a more expensive set, then you might consider trying this type of BTE hearing aids by mail.

Some sellers of hearing aids by mail expect to deal with hearing professionals. These vendors sell products that usually run the buyer into the thousands for a fraction of the cost. The Siemens Intuis is now being offered for a slim $499, while its retail value is around $1800. It is equipped with directional microphones, an auto phone device, and technology that reduce noise and feedback. It is a totally digital aid. There is a similar deal offered in another brand of hearing aid that has similar features. This one lists for $2200 and sells on E-Bay for a mere $399.

It may be to your advantage to buy BTE hearing aids by mail. It is always in your best interest to explore the possibilities. Just remember to find out what it is that you are actually getting for your money. After all, a few hundred dollars spent sounds a lot better than a few thousand, but if the hearing aids aren't what they claim to be, it may be a few hundred dollars wasted. And, who needs that?

Have You Heard Of Beltone Hearing Aids?

Your outside ear is really only there to collect and concentrate sound waves, which vibrate the air in your auditory canal. Air passes the vibration to the eardrum. The hammer bone, inside, is attached to the anvil and stirrup bones, which vibrate the oval window and the round window. This causes fluid to move in the cochlea, which encloses the Organ of Corti. This organ is covered with thousands of tiny hair cells which bring about chemical changes that change electrical potential to create nerve impulses. As you can tell, that little ear on the side of your head is just the beginning of the hearing process, which is a complex bodily instrument! There's more to the hearing process that what was just explained, and the Beltone company has known this for many years.

Beltone hearing aids have been around for at least 67 years, starting in 1940. Their models of digital hearing aids are of a wide variety. The shell styles include Beltone One!, (which is a mini behind-the-ear hearing aid), Beltone Corus, Beltone Linq, Beltone Access, Beltone Edge, Beltone Mira, Beltone Arca, Invisa (in the canal), Petite (in the canal), and the Opera Plus (in the canal).

Beltone has helped countless generations and brought hope and encouragement to many families and individuals who have relied upon their services. They provide other needs besides hearing aids, such as amplified cordless phones, loud alarm clocks, Blue tooth ear sets ($145), neckloops ($150), phone modules ($50), and personal listening systems ($170-$200).

Beltone's listening systems help you hear in public places such as theaters. It can be hard to hear in public places even when you aren't hearing challenged. But those who are were limited for a long time to reading lips and interpreting actions when attending theaters, concerts, and other public events. This has caused them to miss out on much of the understanding they needed for proper processing of the information presented to the audience.

Hearing impaired people were also challenged in the way of waking up in the mornings, even with hearing aids. Many people don't feel a need to sleep with their aids, but when they did have to; they found the older aids uncomfortable for night time relaxation. A timer would be put on an overhead light so that when the light came on, the person would be awakened by the

Hearing Aids Inside Out

brightness. This wouldn't work for the person who can sleep through anything! Even so, the timers couldn't be taken on trips. Wake up calls wouldn't help since the person couldn't hear the phone or a knock on the door. But there are devices now that vibrate, like Beltone's wake and shake alarm clock, which sells for $70. It incorporates a vibration and a flashing strobe that comes on upon the time the alarm is set.

Beltone reaches as far as New England, Canada, and all across the United States; although, one drawback to finding a Beltone representative might be with the challenge of availability in small areas.

Batteries for hearing aids are sold by Beltone, but you can also find them many times in stores. Pharmacies usually carry hearing aid batteries. Typical name brand batteries can sell in a package of 4 for $6. Eco-Gold batteries sell in a package of 6 for $6. You can even order batteries from AARP magazines. They usually sell in bigger bundles than in a store, such as 42 for $25, and offer a refund on the unopened packages if you aren't happy with the product.

How Phonak Hearing Aids Make Listening Easy

Paying attention to your surroundings at all times isn't easy for anyone. It's even harder for those with hearing deficits. Sounds seem muffled or far away. Voices are indecipherable. Furthermore, some hearing aids amplify all sounds, even the ones that are just distracting. Phonak hearing aids can make listening easier for those with hearing loss.

Phonak hearing aids come with different levels of technology. Analog is the least advanced. These are manually adjusted and do not accommodate themselves to a person's preferences automatically. They just receive sound, amplify it, and send it to the ear.

Digitally programmable, also known as analog programmable, is a type that is actually an analog device that can be programmed by using computer software. This allows for some of the advantages of a digital Phonak hearing aid, such as preprogrammed settings, without the expense of a digital.

The digital Phonak hearing aids are where Phonak really shines. With digital technology, it is possible to acquire a hearing aid that is suited to your own personal preferences. This process begins with the fitting, but it doesn't end there.

As you use your Phonak hearing aids you will naturally set the volume as you see fit for the way the setting around you sounds. You will adjust it differently in a crowded football stadium than you will in the relative quiet of your own back porch. After awhile, the Self Learning technology will adapt to the way you do things and will begin to take over the volume adjustments.

Self Logging in you Phonak hearing aids will store information about your choices for use by your audiologist. Then, there is the AutoPilot feature. This element of the hearing aid will automatically change to any of several preset adjustments. The SurroundZoom feature diminishes sounds you'd rather not hear in the background.

Phonak hearing aids offer a version of their aids called the microPower. It is tiny. It only weighs about 2 grams. It is also powerful enough for people with greater hearing loss, because it is essentially a behind the ear, BTE, hearing aid. Its tiny speaker rests in the ear canal. As with other BTE's the speaker and microphone are separate from the speaker and rest behind and on the ear. The tubing they are connected with in this case is extremely small. In fact, all the microStyle hearing aids are similar in size of both the case of the hearing aids and of the tubing. They are also very lightweight.

Phonak hearing aids come in the usual styles. There are ITE, in the ear, hearing aids. These are fine for hearing loss that is not too severe. The BTE, behind the ear, aids are more appropriate for such user with any treatable level of hearing loss and also for children.

Neither Phonak hearing aids nor any other hearing aids are capable of giving your hearing back the way it was before you suffered hearing loss. But, they can make it easier to hear and understand the world around you. With that goal in mind, the use of Phonak hearing aids is worth exploring.

Siemens Artis Hearing Aids May Be The Solution For You

When you are trying to choose the right hearing aid, you may be overwhelmed by the choices on the market. Siemens is one of the top hearing aid companies that want to help the hearing impaired with their outstanding products. A hearing consultant can help you narrow the many choices Siemens offers.

You'll often hear the term 'occlusion' when learning about hearing aids. This means something which blocks the passage. Like some hearing aids that make you feel like you have a big cotton ball stuffed in your ear, occlusion can make you more aware that you have a hearing loss. If you've ever gone under water and tried to hear someone speaking to you who is still above water, you can understand occlusion. You shouldn't feel intimidated by the big terms used when discussing hearing aids or hearing loss. The person who is helping you should be willing to break the terms into more acceptable explanations so you won't walk away feeling like you just don't get it.

Siemens offers aids with digital noise management, speech enhancement, special feedback management, wind noise reduction, trial periods, and ear-to-ear aids. There are 4 types of Artis aids alone---the BTE (behind the ear), the ITE (in the ear), the ITC (in the canal) and the CIC (completely in canal). These can be found for $1600.

A hearing aid is not simply to allow you to hear. It must also monitor, filter, clarify, receive, and control loudness. For many years, people who needed aids in both aids faced additional challenges. Siemens aids can ease that situation as well. If your ears were damaged because of an unhealthy exposure to loud noise on a constant and regular basis, damage to both ears is often the case. Two aids must be able to function well together rather than as 2 separate units for the best performance. The ones Siemens makes are meant to compliment each other and work as a team. The Artis e2e can be found for $1500. Although with this aid, you do have the control to make manual adjustments, they work in sync. A remote control further aids your adjustment capabilities. It can work with only one aid or with an aid in each ear.

The Siemens Artis 2 Life sells for $1100. Feedback is stopped before it happens so there's no uncomfortable squealing whistle to scare those around you. A high pitched sound breaking through the air suddenly can keep a person on edge if it happens often. The Artis 2 Life has an adaptive directional microphone to help you get the most out of the system. If also offers wind screen and automatically adjusts for telephone usage. Battery life is 120 hours.

The Siemens Artis S sells for $1600. The pocket remote is optional and has readouts for volume, program number, and battery life (a whopping 190 hours!). This aid is for mild to moderate loss.

Siemens also offers Artis hearing aids as a full shell, half shell, canal, mini canal, and CIC at price ranges from $1350 to $1450. All are available with the remote control option for $150.

The Benefits Of Starkey Hearing Aids

Hearing aids have become so much more technologically advanced that they even include devices which allow the users to listen to IPODS! In-line telephone amplifiers can be carried on trips to help with hotel phone use. There are devices the hearing impaired can take to movie theaters to help them hear the movie while blocking out the unnecessary background noises.

One of the popular companies that seem to be on top with their innovating products that carry users into the future is Starkey. They have aids that will appeal to children as well as adults. If your child is embarrassed at the thought of having to learn to use a hearing aid, their feelings should be respected. Starkey can help ease the situation. They've taken the care and the time to help equip children around the world.

It may help to have the child first try the hearing device at home for a short while before having them use it at school. They must become accustomed to the feel of the aid and may need help feeling less self-conscious about using an aid. They'll have to be taught the proper care, handling, storage, and not to share the aid with other curious children. Try finding other children who also wear a hearing aid who may be willing to communicate with your child. Children's care facilities, children's hospitals, other adults who wear hearing aids... all have potential for a support system for your child.

The Starkey Hearing Foundation has provided over 20,000 aids to people who needed help acquiring them. It's located in Minnesota, but reaches far beyond with its assistance. Starkey has a program called StarKids, which is a help to parents and children as they learn about hearing aids. You may need the hearing aid yourself and will want to help your child understand your device better.

Starkey Laboratories used to be a small ear mold company until William F. Austin took an interest in it. He merged it with his own company, which repaired hearing devices. Now there are Starkey facilities in more than 24 countries, with subsidiary companies in California and Minnesota. You may have heard of Audibel, Micro-Tech, and Nu-Ear.

Hearing Aids Inside Out

Starkey has aids with helpful features that include a diagnostic tool that provides a performance report of the hearing aid. It will actually remind you when it's time for your follow-up visit! If you're interested in this particular aid, it's called the Destiny 1600 and runs around $2400. Keep in mind that the best hearing aid features will cost more. If you just want the basics, Starkey has those as well.

For models like the Davinci PSP line, the cost can be as much as $2200. The Sierra line sells for $1700. Starkey's Axent line sells for $2100. The Aspect Xtra sells for $2100. There are lower cost Starkey products, such as the Starkey A13 MPT-1 and the Starkey A13 Sequel MMP BTE-1. Aids along this line can run anywhere from $570 to $1400.

A few of the famous people who have been associated with the Starkey name are Ronald Reagan, Elton John, and Jay Leno.

What To Look For In Inexpensive Hearing Aids

With hearing aids costing thousands of dollars each in some cases, it's easy to become discouraged. It's easy to give up and say to yourself that you'll just have to learn to live with not being able to hear. Maybe you can learn to lip read, you think. But, what if you can find hearing aids that you can afford? Maybe you can. You just need to know what to look for in inexpensive hearing aids.

There are some devices that send the sound to your ear with very little processing except a bit of amplification. Some of these are not even sold as hearing aids, but are sold to hunters who want to be able to hear wildlife noises very well. These are rightfully called listening devices. They do not meet FDA guidelines that describe what constitutes a hearing aid. At prices usually under $20 each, they claim to be inexpensive hearing aids, but they are not considered by most to be hearing aids at all.

Watch out for companies that insist on you signing a waiver of medical care before they will send you your hearing aids. These companies do not expect to go through a hearing professional. If that's what you want, then so be it. Just make sure you are aware of the consequences of this decision. If you have a medical condition that is causing your hearing loss, it might be serious and it might be better if you had it checked out. But, that is your call. Maybe this is the way you want to go about getting inexpensive hearing aids.

Your best bet is to look for deals on well-known brands and models of hearing aids. These can be found at better prices than the manufacturer offers, if you look on the internet. Just make sure you are comparing the exact same brand names and models of hearing aids to the same inexpensive hearing aids you have found. Also, make sure that they are new and have a warranty. Find out about trial periods and return policies. If you go through your ENT doctor, you will find that you will be given a rather long trial period. At any time during this period, you can bring the hearing aids back for a full refund minus a very small restocking fee. The same policy does not go for all sellers, especially internet sellers.

Another thing to look for is how the inexpensive hearing aids are fitted, both in physical conformity to your ear canal and in volume, frequency, and sound memories. Some inexpensive hearing aids are BTE hearing aids that come with a universal ear mold to start you off. They also come with the capability of providing a custom fitted ear mold by taking the aid to your audiologist.

Some inexpensive hearing aids are designed for you to do the programming of the hearing aid yourself with the help of computer software. You have to decide if you are up to that challenge if you choose a package like this.

Some of these inexpensive hearing aids can be fitted through an ENT doctor and some are done without any doctor. Whatever you choose to do about your hearing problems, look for reliable yet inexpensive hearing aids for the solution.

What You Need To Know About To Compare Hearing Aids

You have just realized you have hearing loss. Or, you have recently gained the ability to do something about it. Now you have to sort through all the different styles, models, and manufacturers to find the right ones for you. You can no doubt get some help from your audiologist, but if you want to be an informed consumer, you will want to learn to compare hearing aids for yourself.

When you do compare hearing aids, the first question is whether you want to get analog or digital hearing aids. Analog are the least expensive by far. These hearing aids simply receive a signal from a microphone, amplify it, and send the louder sound on to the ear. It's as simple as that.

There is a middle ground between analog and digital. These are sometimes called digital programmable, although they are not 100 percent digital, or they are called analog programmable. The idea here is that it is indeed an analog hearing aid. It just has the advantage of a certain amount of customization in programming through the use of computer software. This can give you a variety of settings you can manually switch to accommodate your listening preferences in different listening situations. The settings can be changed by reprogramming at any time. When you compare hearing aids, these are more expensive than the regular analog ones, but less so than fully digital ones.

Fully digital hearing aids are the most expensive, and when you compare hearing aids you will find many reasons why this is so. The difference in sound quality is like the difference you get when you go to digital music recordings from old fashioned record albums. This is done through DSP, or digital signal processing.

There are differences in the programming as well. One thing to notice when you compare hearing aids is how many channels or bands it has. This is important because if your hearing loss is not the same for all frequencies, you will want different frequencies adjusted differently. Some people may only need a couple of bands while others may need several.

Hearing Aids Inside Out

It is also nice to know if a hearing aid has directional microphones. If it does, there are two microphones that emphasize sounds in front of you rather than behind you. Some models have a switch so that you can turn this feature on and off.

Another way to compare hearing aids is by taking into account how many preset programs there are to switch between. You might want different programs for different aspects of your life, like home and work environments, and the surroundings at your favorite free time activities.

Compare hearing aids by noting which ones are "smart" hearing aids. These have the capability to learn your preferences by the way you use them when you get them. These are easy to operate because, after awhile, the hearing aid automatically sets itself the way you usually set it yourself. Other features are reduced feedback and wind noise, and the ability to use the device with phones or even mobile phones.

In the end, you will probably talk it over with your audiologist before you make your final decision. It's nice to go in to that talk armed with some facts of your own. That is why it's in your best interest to compare hearing aids yourself.

What You Should Know About Digital Hearing Aids

There are digital hearing aids available without a doctor's prescription or testing. Some of the aids you can buy that go in the ear canal are digi-ears, which range from $300 to $700 and have various additions. They're versatile to fit either ear, so if you bought two of the same type, you wouldn't have to worry about which aid would fit each ear if you got confused.

Many different digital hearing aids are available. Some of them include a two channel value aid, which is a low cost aid, a mid-level four channel aid that provides feedback reduction and a speech amplifier, and the best level (also a four channel aid), which offers echo suppression and layered noise reduction. All of these aids come with a wax remover. (Wax seems to be a problem for hearing aid wearers and must be kept to a minimum for the best reception.)

You may want a carrying case for your digital hearing aid, to keep it safe by the bedside or in the nightstand while you sleep. The carrying case can help protect it from insects or dust or even a naughty cat who likes to knock things off furniture! Keeping your digital aid clean and dry is important for proper function and long-lasting use.

Digital aids use microprocessors to process sound for you to hear and should adjust volume according to sound levels. There are different frequency levels an aid must allow for; each level will have its own amount of hearing loss. This makes the correct purchase of an aid even more important. An ill fit, improper adjustment, or neglect to the proper levels you will need help with are reasons you should be properly tested and should use a professional to help you choose the right aid for you. Your lifestyle and budget are, of course, two other important factors to consider. You'll want to work with a quality hearing aid supplier, purchase an aid made by a reputable company, and go through the proper medical channels to help you make the best decision.

Almost any company that sells hearing aids will now have digital aids available for purchase. Digital aids can reduce or eliminate feedback while the person wears them. They have gain processing, which reduces microphone noise and environmental sounds. Speech recognition is more accurate with less annoying interruptions to filter through to hear what someone is saying. If you've ever held a large seashell up to your ear, you should recall the loud white noise it makes. Suppose you had to walk around every day with that noise in your ear, making it hard to decipher what anyone is trying to tell you at any time of the day or night. Digital aids have been improved to overcome that type of obstacle. They have been improved to help cut down on the equipment a person used to be burdened with when wearing a hearing aid. Digital aids are more easily adjusted with more built-in capabilities than ever before. They even include signal generators to increase accuracy with your fittings.

Would You Take A Chance On A Cheap Hearing Aid?

One of the most frustrating things for a hearing impaired person to deal with is a cheap hearing aid. To have a hearing problem can be frustrating in itself, but to have to continually fight with a malfunctioning or low quality hearing aid is adding insult to injury. Poor workmanship or cheap parts make hearing a nightmare for the hearing impaired. It is understandable that some people just can't afford a good quality aid; and insurance companies have long been ornery about helping the hearing impaired. But buying a better quality aid is better in the long run than wasting hard-earned money on several cheap aids that just don't last!

Hearing your car make a noise when starting up or traveling may be crucial to your engine being repaired properly and may keep you from having an accident. Hearing a vehicle approach may save your life or the life of a small child who is with you. Hearing your child scream for help may be what keeps them from being injured further or kidnapped by a stranger. Hearing the phone ring, hearing a baby cry, hearing a warning to keep you out of danger or hearing an animal approach could all be important life happenings that you'd miss should you choose to buy a cheap hearing aid. Suppose you were at an important event and your child or grandchild was counting on you to hear them sing or to hear their important part in a play? If your cheap aid is inhibiting your lifestyle, maybe it would be well worth the investment to treat yourself (and your family) to a quality hearing aid.

Unfortunately, not all dealers of hearing aids will have your best interests at heart when trying to sell you a hearing aid. Should you have the little voice inside trying to warn you about a shady deal, it pays to listen to it. The hearing aid should be an important step to changing your life for the better. Research the company, ask people who already have hearing aids, and check out the different brands and prices available before deciding to purchase. In other words, shop around, not only for the best aid, but for the best person to help you make your purchase. Ask an audiologist for references. Make sure the person you purchase your aid from is easily available for any future questions, or can tell you the steps you need to take should any problems occur. You should be satisfied that you are getting your questions answered clearly. Ask about warranties and availability of any service or parts and any costs that may be involved. Don't just assume that paying for the aid itself is all the cost you would have to incur.

Hearing Aids Inside Out

Technology has made leaps and bounds when it comes to developing better hearing aids over the years. The hearing aids of today make the older ones from years ago seem like cheap hearing aids. Aids today allow even for whispers in some cases. Cheap aids may lack the proper control over volume adjustment, noise filtering, whistling, and clarity of sound.

Finding The Right Digital Hearing Aids For You

Getting digital hearing aids is something that will improve your hearing greatly, but what kind of hearing aids do you need? Digital are the best out there. With this kind of hearing aid you'll be able to program your hearing aid yourself. It starts with volume control, power and much more. Digital hearing aids are the latest technology on the market for hearing aids. Buying something like this might be just what you need.

Don't let the technology scare you; these hearing aids are very easy to use. The hearing aids can also be programmed when you get them. This will help to get your hearing just right. There is a chance that your hearing might decrease as you get older, with a digital hearing aid you can change the settings to work for you.

You will have to train your digital hearing aid until it is just right. But once you go through this process there is little else you need to do for your hearing aid. Digital hearing aids also make sure that you hear what you need to hear. There will be some background noises, but they will bring the sounds you need to hear up to the foreground. It might take a while to get use to, but once you do you'll be hearing fine.

If you do plan on buying digital hearing aids make sure that you know that they will cost some money. Look around, check online and see what they have to offer. Hearing aids of any kind will be an investment in good hearing. Think about looking at buying the digital hearings aids as something that will last longer then any thing on the market. Also think about you're hearing in the future, the digital hearing aid will change with your hearing need.

Once you decided on getting digital hearing aids make sure you know what the return policy is. Make sure that you know when the date is up on being able to return your hearing aids. You should even talk to the person you bought them from, or the site you bought them from and see if they have any information. Also, don't settle on something you don't like. You will need to make sure you give yourself time to get used to the hearing aids.

Knowing If Your Child Needs Hearing Aids

Sometimes it's not an older adult that needs hearing aids it might be a small child. This could be a hearing problem that started when the child was born or has grown over the years. There are ways to see if your child is not hearing right, these are quick ways to check before you take your child to a doctor.

For a newborn, if your child doesn't waken at loud noises, calm down at the sound of your voice. For a few months older, if your child doesn't turn their eyes toward you, smile when spoke to, notice rattles or other noise making noise toys. For a year or older they should be able to say different words, listen to what you are saying, putting words together and even naming few objects.

If any of the problems stated above have occurred with you're child you should take them to you're local doctor right away. Your doctor should be able to tell you what kind of hearing problem you're child has. It might be something as simple as an ear infection or something that will require hearing aids.

It would be best to find out if you're child has hearing problems sooner rather then later. This can help you're child get used to having hearing aids. Researching hearing aids can be the fastest way to find what you need to know about the kind of hearing aids for your child. It might be best to look into buying digital hearing aids. These hearing aids are ones that can be changed with hearing needs.

This could save you money from buying other hearing aids down the line. Another way to save money is to look on the Internet for sites that sell hearing aids. If you're looking online for child hearing aids look for a smaller set, these will be smaller to fit into a child's hear. Buying online might turn out to be cheaper then buying hearing aids from a local shop. You should know the return policies if you go with this route.

Remember that it is the right course of action that you take your child to a doctor before you think of buying any hearing aids. This will save you money and keep you're child's hearing in top shape.

Digital Hearing Aids And Other Types

If you are just researching about hearing aids then you should know what kind of hearing aids that you can find. There are many out there and if you are buying hearing aids online it will be different from buying hearing aids in a store. The one plus thing about this is that most of the hearing aids sites online will give you a buyer's guide.

Another thing to know is what kind of hearing aids you can get.

- **In the Ear or ITE**

These hearing aids are they kind that fit in the outer ear. They are used for a wide range of hearing loss. This type of hearing aid is larger then others. ITE hearing aids can be used around technology also.

- **Behind the Ear or BTE**

These hearing aids are worn behind the ear. Because these are larger they might be able to help you pick up small sounds.

- **CompletelyintheCanalorCIC**

This hearing aid fits down into the canal of the ear and you won't be able to see it. Because of how small this hearing aid is it might not be the right choice for people with severe hearing loss.

- **In the Canal or ITC**

These are similar to CIC but this type is larger and doesn't fit right into the ear canal.

With so many choices to pick from you need to take time and decide what you need to use for you. Knowing that you have a hearing problem is the first step. Looking online for information on hearing aids will help you deicide what kind of hearing help you need.

If you do want to buy your hearing aids online and don't have a computer then you can ask a friend or a son, daughter. They'll be able to help you find what you are looking for online and find information that you need.

From there you can find the type of hearing aid you need online and buy right then. Make sure that you know the site you are buying from has a return policy or a buyer's guide. Make sure that you don't settle on the first hearing aid you buy online. You want to find something that is comfortable and makes your hearing better.

Differences Between Digital Hearing Aids And Others

Know about the technology that will be in the hearing aids that you are thinking of buying or going to buy. Knowing what goes into your hearing aids might help you decide what you are going to buy.

There are a lot of different technologies that are used in hearing aids. Knowing what your hearing aid will have inside it might help you decide before you buy.

- **Analog or traditional**

Most of the hearing aids use analog technology to amplify sounds. There is one problem with this type of technology; all the sounds are amplified at the same time. Some people have trouble trying to work around all the noise. If this is the case you can have the hearing aid built to you're needs. Also, analog hearing aids are cheaper then others.

- **Programmable Hearing Aids**

These types of hearing aids are a skip up from the analog system. This is because they can be adjusted and programmed. These hearing aids will come with more then one setting. Also some might even have controls that you can use to change the setting while you are in different surroundings.

- **Digital**

This type is the most advanced of the hearing aids. Using one or more microchip they convert the analog sounds to a digital signal. This type is also easier for sounds to be separated into channels. Remember though that this type of hearing aids is the expensive type.

With the three types above you can pick what kind you want to buy. With each one you'll have to decide what could work for you. From how large you want the hearing aid to the how you want your hearing aid to work.

Hearing Aids Inside Out

Choices the technology that you want is one of the steps. If you are buying online then you should be able to find more information on the site you chose to buy your hearing aids from. Check the site out before you decide to place you're order. See if they have a return policy or a buyer's guide. This will help you get the best hearing aid that you need.

Make sure that you don't settle on something that you don't like. You've paid money to get good hearing aids, make sure that you get your money out of what you've bought.

Knowing When It's Time For Hearing Aids

Knowing that you need a hearing aid is one of the battles of wanting to hear well. Answering a simple list of questions will be enough to know if you do having hearing loss.

- Ifsoundsorspeechismuffled.
- Ifyoucan'tunderstandwords.Moresoifyou'reinalargeroomandcanonlyhear background noise.
- Askingpeopleyoutalkwithtorepeatwhattheysay,ortoslowdownwhentheyaretalking. • TurningupthevolumeforyourTVormusic.

There is a possibility that you have something else wrong with just hearing loss. There are many reasons for sudden hearing loss. Knowing if you have one of these problems might stop you from having to buy hearing aids.

- Earwax blockage
- Ear infection
- Airplane ear
- Swimmer's ear
- Returned eardrum

Each one of these can be seen and fixed by seeing a doctor. Looking up any of these ear problems for more information might give you the knowledge you need to know if you have an ear problem or actual hearing loss.

The best way to find out if you have a hearing problem is to see a doctor. They'll be able to make sure that you get the right treatment for the right hearing needs. From here you can see a hearing aid specialist. Or look online and see what you can find online.

Knowing what kind of hearing aid you need. Getting digital hearing aids might be the right option for you once you know that you have hearing loss. With so many hearing aids on the market finding the right one might be difficult. Think of getting hearing aids as an investment to have good hearing.

Thinking this way you should look into getting something that will last and be able to change with your hearing. With new technology digital hearing aids are the best thing on the market to buy. They'll be able to change with your hearing needs over the years.

Make sure that you look around before you buy, from looking online to see what companies have to offer. Make sure that you read all the information for any company you buy from. Know what you want and how much you are willing to spend for it.

Do You Have The Proper Hearing Aids?

If you have hearing aids already and have decided that it is time for new hearing aids you should think about looking into to digital hearing aids. These types of hearing aids are the newest kind that you can find on the market. They can also change with your hearing needs.

You should make sure that you go to your doctor before getting new hearing aids. Your doctor should know what kind of hearing aids you need and if you need a different type. This will be something that you might have to do before you buy new hearing aids.

Replacing your hearing aids after so many years might seem to be a hassle, but with the new technology that has came out. Thinking of replacing your hearing aids might be a great idea. Looking into or buying digital hearing might worth looking into.

They will be expensive but will last you a long time. They'll also be able to change with you're hearing needs. This will save you from having to buy another pair a few years later. Being able to change the volume of your digital hearing aid is something that will help you hear better.

One idea to think of when looking for digital hearing aids is to look online. These days you can find anything online. Buying hearing aids over an Internet site might be easier then you think. Also they might be cheaper then buying them from a store in your town. If you don't have a computer ask a friend, most libraries have computers with an Internet connection, or ask a family member.

Once you find a site you like then you can look into the site history. Learn about the return policies. From there you can also look at other sites and compare prices of what kind of hearing aid you need. If you know what you want in a hearing aid then you can find. This will narrow you're search for your hearing aids online.

Make sure that you get what you want. Don't buy the first thing you find, look around. Compare other items to what you have found. Doing this you should find the best digital hearing aid for the best price. This will be the best way to get your hearing back.

Digital Hearing Aids For Older Parents

If you have older parents that might have hearing problems it might be time to look into getting hearing aids for them. With technology you can find great hearing aids for not that much. Looking online can help you decide what kind of hearing aids will be the best kind.

Or if you don't know if your parents need hearing aids then you should look for the signs. Are they having a hard time understanding words? Do they turn the volume up loud for the TV or play music loudly? To they have a hard time following a conversation in a noisy room? This is the case for older people, but in some cases it might be another matter, you should see if you can get a hold of a doctor and set an appointment up.

Spending more money for a digital set of hearing aids might be just what you are looking for. These are the highest technology that hearing aids have. Don't worry if your parents aren't technologically advanced, digital hearing aids are made to be easy to use and wear.

With digital hearing aids you are able to change the settings if you're hearing gets worse. It might be best to see if your parents have a doctor, if not see if you can set up an appointment for hearing. This will help your parents know if they do need hearing aids.

These days you can even find hearing aids to buy online. You might find that this is a cheaper route to go then to buy from someone in town. Make sure that you check the sites out that you look at. Compare prices from each site that you find. From there you can easily buy online. Make sure that you know what the sites return policy is in case the hearing aids don't work or are wrong.

If your parents still aren't sure if they want hearing aids, they might think differently after they've tried a few for a little while. It might be something that they need to try for themselves. That or you can give them information on hearing aids and see if they want to buy them their selves. Either way, buying hearing aids will make hearing much easier.

Pros And Cons Of Digital Hearing Aids

If you're thinking about getting hearing aids you might want to think about the pros and cons of getting hearing aids. The first pro you can think about is knowing that you'll be able to hear better then you have in a while. Maybe you don't think that hearing aids are going to help you.

With the technology that hearing aids are made with these days the help in hearing you'll be able to receive will be very shocking. Though with so many hearing aids on the market what kind of hearing aids will be the best for you? If you do plan on spending a fair sum of money and then look into something that will last a long time.

The best technology for hearing aids right now is the digital hearing aids. These can be changed with you're hearing needs, another pro that you can consider. Buying something that will be able to change over with your hearing needs is something that will save you money in the long run.

Another pro is the fact that you can now use the Internet to compare prices of what you're willing to spend. There is a down side to using the internet, that being not being able to get a hold of a computer or a computer with the Internet. This can be easily solved from asking a family member or seeing if your town has a computer café.

Another con can be to worry about getting something that is considered technologically advanced. Digital hearing aids have been made to be easy to use. From here you might look at other pro and cons that you have thought of, price might be one, but if you spend a little extra you can have something that will last longer and be able to change with you're hearing needs.

Pros and cons aside think of what you need in a hearing aid, from a digital one to something that is a different type of technology. Learn about what you are planning to buy before you do is another way to make a pro and con list. Anything kind of research can help in deciding if you want to buy digital hearing aids. Writing down a pro and con list is just one of the ways to start with.

Basic Knowledge Of Digital Hearing Aids

If you're looking into getting digital hearing aids then you should know what kind of hearing aids you are getting. Knowing about what you are buying will help you in the long run of buying you're digital hearing aids. There are many types on the market and you should find something that works for you. here are a few you can read about.

- **Advance signal processing**

This type of hearing aid adjusts the amount of sound that the hearing aid provides from how much sound the microphone inside the hearing aid is picking up. like most digital hearing aids this type also has capitally to let users hear while in noisy rooms.

- **Multi-Channel Capability**

Digital hearing aids have more then one frequency. This helps the hearing aid hear different pitched sounds; this will help the user wearing the hearing aid. This also provides more flexibility to help meet the user needs.

- **Multi-Memory Capability**

Some digital hearing aids have a memory. This allows the storage of more then one frequencies program. This lets the user pick from different programs by pressing a button on the hearing aid.

- **Noise reduction capability**

Some digital hearing aids are made to reduce background noise when heard. This will help with hearing in a large room or a crowded meeting and more.

Not all hearing aids can completely block out all background noise. Though now most digital hearing aids can determine between background noise and normal speech. Also when thinking of getting hearings, one thing to know is that you have a hearing aid that can change with you're needs of hearing.

There is one down side with the digital hearing aids, they do cost money. But if you plan on putting money into getting hearing aids, think of placing some extra with the money you have and get the digital hearing aids. Buying a set of digital hearing aids can be a great investment that can change with you're hearing needs over time. This will cut down on the need to buy new hearing aids over time. Looking online can also cut down the price of you're digital hearing aids. From here you can deicide if it will be worth the extra money to buy digital hearing aids.

Digital Hearing Aids Versus Analog

Thinking about getting hearing aids is something that you should know about before you plan to buy. The one thing you need to decide on is what kind of hearing aid you want to buy. You should look at all kinds before you decide on one type of hearing aid. Knowing what you plan on buying is another way you can make sure that you have the best kind of hearing aids.

There are two different types of hearing aids on the market, analog hearing aids and digital hearing aids. Each of these are great hearing aids, these hearing aids all have pros and cons. Look at each of them it will be up to you to decide what type of hearing aids are right for you.

Analog hearing aids to cost less then digital hearing aids. Batteries also last longer in analog hearing aids. These are pros for the analog hearing aid. As for digital hearing aids you can have the sound changed without having to ship the hearing aids back to the manufacturer. Sound can also be adjusted to fit your likes and dislikes.

There are other types of hearing aids also you can look into, like true digital hearing aids. Some advantages for this type of hearing aids are noise reduction; this will help cut down on background noise. This type of hearing aid will have multiple memories for different hearing needs. This type also has the greatest ability to be adjusted by you.

What kind of hearing aid is up to you in the long run? You should look into each type of hearing aids and decide what is best for you. Knowing that analog might be cheaper might not be the best route to go. Spending extra money to buy digital will give you hearing aids that can change with your hearing needs.

Researching what type of hearing aid you want even farther can help you decide. From what brands are the best to where is the best place to buy hearing aids. With the Internet you can find a great wealth of extra information. Also you can find sites online that you can buy your hearings aids from, this can be cheaper then finding a company in your city.

Telecoil Hearing Aids

A very useful feature found in most behind the ear hearing aids and some in the ear hearing aids is the telecoil. It's also sometimes known as a t-switch or t-coil. Telecoils allow the hearing aid to receive signals from different electronic sources. They can provide better sound quality and eliminate background noise in certain situations. Telecoils can be used with some telephones, FM radio systems and public address systems.

A telecoil consists of wire wrapped around a metal core. This allows a telecoil to produce through induction an electrical signal when in the presence of an electromagnetic field. Thus telecoils will pick up magnetic signals like a microphone picks up a sound signal. The telecoil will bypass the hearing aid's microphone and transmit this signal directly to the hearing aid's processing circuits for amplification.

The telecoil was originally designed to be used with old-style telephones. This is where the name telecoil comes from. These phones produced a strong magnetic field from the speakers in the ear piece. The telecoil would allow its user to hear the telephone better, as it would allow the user to not amplify the background noise.

Newer phones do not produce the same strong magnetic fields as older phones. However, most phones are designated as hearing aid compatible, or HAC. This means that they can produce the signals needed for the telecoil to work properly. In addition, many movie theaters, auditoriums, and sports stadiums provide assistive listening systems to those patrons that require them. These generally take the form of hearing aid compatible headsets or receivers which can be borrowed by those who need them.

There are also a series of loop devices that can produce the magnetic fields needed by telecoils. They are generally hooked directly into a sound source like a television, radio or PA system. The three types of loop devices are room loops, neck loops, and silhouettes. Room loops are built into a room, either in the ceiling, floor or baseboards. The magnetic signal they produce can be used by everyone in the room, making them suitable for areas where there are many hearing aid users, like a church or nursing home. A neck loop and a silhouette are both single user devices, the neck loop being the size of a necklace, and the silhouette being even smaller and designed to fit behind the ear.

The advantage of a telecoil is that you can bypass the microphone on your hearing aid and therefore minimize the effect of background noise. Telecoils made it possible for hearing aid users to hear important communication in difficult situations, like a crowded theater.

Types Of Hearing Aids

A hearing aid is a device that helps someone who has trouble hearing. Hearing aids today are electronic instruments that receive and amplify sounds. The first hearing aids are now known as body worn aids. They are bulky instruments about the size of a deck of cards that are designed to be carried in a pocket. A wire connects the hearing aid to an earphone. Body worn aids are seldom used anymore, except occasionally in the case of very severe hearing loss.

The most common hearing aid type today is the behind the ear aid, or BTE. A behind the ear hearing aid consists of a case that clips behind the ear and is connected directly by plastic sound tubes to a custom molded earpiece. BTE's are used for a wide range of hearing losses. Behind the ear hearing aids generally have a larger battery than other types of hearing aids, allowing them to be more powerful and have a longer life.

With improved technology and miniaturization of electronics, the next generation of hearing aids, in the ear or ITE, became possible. These aids fit in the outer ear bowl. ITE's can be visible to the casual observer. They are also the largest of the custom made styles, and are often the most comfortable, cheapest and simplest to use. Smaller that the in the ear hearing aid is the in the canal, or ITC hearing aid. These aids are usually more expensive than ITE's, and are also harder to adjust owing to the small size of the volume wheel. Going even smaller we find the mini canal, or MC hearing aid. These are the smallest hearing aid you can get that still have a volume adjustment wheel.

The tiniest hearing aids made are the completely in the canal, or CIC hearing aids. They fit so deeply into the ear that they require a removal string. CIC's do not usually have manual controls simply because of their size.

Combining some of the attributes of the behind the ear and the completely in the canal hearing aids are the post auricular canal devices. This design physically separates the processor from the earpiece. The small processor fits behind the ear, while the receiver and speaker portion is imbedded in the earpiece which is placed deep in the ear canal.

Choosing a type of hearing aid is usually making a trade-off between size, price and flexibility.

The largest hearing aids used today, the BTE's, are generally the cheapest, most powerful, easiest to adjust and the most durable. However, they are also the most conspicuous. BTE's tend to be the best choice for children, however, owing to their durability and the ability to replace the earpiece as the child grows. Other types of hearing aids would have to be replaced periodically when the child outgrows them.

Hearing Aids In Children

A hearing aid is a device that helps someone who has trouble hearing. Hearing aids today are electronic instruments that receive and amplify sounds. The first hearing aids are now known as body worn aids. They are bulky instruments about the size of a deck of cards that are designed to be carried in a pocket. A wire connects the hearing aid to an earphone. Body worn aids are seldom used anymore, except occasionally in the case of very severe hearing loss.

The most common hearing aid type today is the behind the ear aid, or BTE. A behind the ear hearing aid consists of a case that clips behind the ear and is connected directly by plastic sound tubes to a custom molded earpiece. BTE's are used for a wide range of hearing losses. Behind the ear hearing aids generally have a larger battery than other types of hearing aids, allowing them to be more powerful and have a longer life.

With improved technology and miniaturization of electronics, the next generation of hearing aids, in the ear or ITE, became possible. These aids fit in the outer ear bowl. ITE's can be visible to the casual observer. They are also the largest of the custom made styles, and are often the most comfortable, cheapest and simplest to use. Smaller that the in the ear hearing aid is the in the canal, or ITC hearing aid. These aids are usually more expensive than ITE's, and are also harder to adjust owing to the small size of the volume wheel. Going even smaller we find the mini canal, or MC hearing aid. These are the smallest hearing aid you can get that still have a volume adjustment wheel.

The tiniest hearing aids made are the completely in the canal, or CIC hearing aids. They fit so deeply into the ear that they require a removal string. CIC's do not usually have manual controls simply because of their size.

Combining some of the attributes of the behind the ear and the completely in the canal hearing aids are the post auricular canal devices. This design physically separates the processor from the earpiece. The small processor fits behind the ear, while the receiver and speaker portion is imbedded in the earpiece which is placed deep in the ear canal.

Choosing a type of hearing aid is usually making a trade-off between size, price and flexibility.

The largest hearing aids used today, the BTE's, are generally the cheapest, most powerful, easiest to adjust and the most durable. However, they are also the most conspicuous. BTE's tend to be the best choice for children, however, owing to their durability and the ability to replace the earpiece as the child grows. Other types of hearing aids would have to be replaced periodically when the child outgrows them.

Do You Need Hearing Aids?

If you suspect you have hearing loss you need to visit your family doctor. They can check for signs of a medical condition that would affect your hearing. Of the two types of hearing loss, conductive and sensorineural, it is sensorineural hearing loss that is generally corrected with a hearing aid. Your doctor will examine your ear with an instrument called an otoscope. With an otoscope, your doctor can see if there are any abnormalities in your ear canal or eardrum. The next step is to conduct a full hearing test. One portion of this test is the pure tone testing, which measures how well you hear different frequencies. You will be asked to listen to a series of tones at various volumes, and to indicate when you hear them. Each ear will be tested separately. Another type of pure tone tests involves the placement of a small bone conductor behind your ear, which allows sound waves to be transmitted directly to the cochlea of the inner ear, bypassing the middle and outer ear.

After the pure tone tests, you most likely will have to take a series of speech tests. Here you will be asked to detect and understand speech. You will hear a series of words that you will be asked to repeat. The words will vary in intensity and length. An impedance test is used to measure the transmission of sound through the middle ear. An audiologist will check this by placing a probe in your ear and measuring the transmission of various tones and frequencies at different air pressures.

The results of a hearing test are usually presented in a chart known as an audiogram. Your audiologist will explain this chart to you. It will show your perception of different frequencies, and compares that with the expected values. An audiogram is a useful tool in measuring the progress of hearing loss over time. An audiogram will present the results in terms of decibels. A decibel is a logarithmic measure of sound intensity. Zero decibels is defined as the intensity that a normal person can hear fifty percent of the time. A normal conversation occurs at about forty five decibels, and one hundred and twenty decibels is the noise a 747 would make while taking off.

Shopping For Hearing Aids

The first thing to do if you suspect you have hearing loss is to see your family doctor. They can check your ears for signs of blockage or infection. If neither is present, they may send you to either an otolaryngologist or an audiologist. An otolaryngologist is an ear, nose and throat doctor, and can best diagnose medical problems with your ears. An audiologist is a professional with an advanced degree. They specialize in testing for hearing loss and hearing aid fitting. It is also possible to obtain a hearing aid directly from a hearing aid dealer or consultant. They will be trained to test for hearing loss, and to fit and sell hearing aids.

The next step is to get a full hearing test. This should consists of several different tests, including the lowest sound you can hear, how well you can hear speech in different environments, and how well you tolerate loud noises. Your perception of different tones or frequencies should also be measured.

You should discuss with your doctor or audiologist whether a hearing aid is the best solution for you, or whether it is possible to correct your hearing loss through surgery.

Next you'll want to select the hearing aid that is right for you. Make sure you investigate the three main styles of hearing aids (BTE, ITE, and CIC). Most hearing aid companies offer a trial period, so don't be hesitant to try more than one aid. You will want to choose a hearing aid that is both comfortable and will most effectively improve your hearing. Learn what features are available with the different hearing aids; in particular telecoil is a useful feature that you should seriously consider. You may want to ask about the possibility of direct audio input which would allow you to use assistive listening devices which can be found in some schools, movies theatres and other public auditoriums.

Itisimportanttounderstandallthecostsofahearingaid,includingbatteriesandrepairs. You may end up going through batteries quite frequently, so remember to compare expected battery life with the price per battery. At this time it is also important to learn what the warranty covers, and for how long. It may be worth it to extend the warranty.

A new hearing aid can be a disorienting experience. Become familiar with your hearing aid.

Hearing Aids Inside Out

Make sure you are comfortable putting in and taking out the aid, adjusting the volume control, and replacing the batteries before you leave the audiologist. A common complaint of new hearing aid users is that their own voices may sound too loud. This usually takes some time to get used to. Another problem is feedback, where your hearing aid produces a whistle. This is caused by the fit of the hearing aid or by the buildup of earwax or fluid. You will need to see your audiologist for adjustments.

Maintaining Your Hearing Aids

In order to get a long and productive life from your hearing aid, it is very important to maintain it properly. Hearing aids are delicate instruments, and looking after them properly is vital. You will need to know how to clean your hearing aid by removing wax buildup, how to replace and dispose of batteries and how to remove moisture from the aid.

You should put together a kit for maintaining your hearing aids. In this kit you will want a battery tester and spare batteries, silica gel packs and a plastic stethoscope. In addition, if you have a behind the ear hearing aid you will want a forced air ear mold blower. Dead batteries are probably the most common cause of hearing aid malfunction. You will want to replace dead batteries immediately. The spare batteries you have in your kit will be very useful when this occurs. There is nothing worse than been stuck with dead batteries when you have an event to go to! You will want to remember to turn off your hearing aids when you're not using them in order to prolong the battery life. The silica gel packs are used to prevent moisture from getting into your hearing aid while you are not wearing it.

It is generally a good idea to keep hearing aids away from heat and moisture. Avoid using hairspray or other hair care products while wearing your hearing aid. Keep your hearing aid clean by wiping it with a tissue daily. Make sure you check for damage such as cracks, broken parts, clogged openings or moisture.

Every day, check to make sure that your hearing aid is working properly by listening to it through the stethoscope. Vary the volume while doing this to ensure that the sound is clear and strong without any static or unusual sounds. To make sure the hearing aid is producing a clear sound for you, set the hearing aid to a volume where you like to listen through the hearing aid. Ensure that the hearing aid is not cutting in and out.

The only part of a hearing aid that should be washed is the ear mold piece of a behind the ear hearing aid. Gently wash it with a mild detergent or an ear mold cleaning kit. The forced air blower can be used to dry the ear mold more quickly. The plastic tubing should be checked for stiffness and cracks. It will probably need to be replaced every six months or so.

In the ear and smaller hearing aids should be cleaned with a dry tissue and small brush on a daily basis. Do not attempt to wash them with a damp cloth, as this will damage them.

If you are having any problems with your hearing aid, take it back to the dispenser or audiologist to ensure that it is still properly adjusted for you. The hearing aid will be of no use to you if you do not wear it, so it makes sense to properly maintain it.

Improvements To Hearing Aids

Many hearing aids now have directional microphones. These can be a major improvement in areas with a lot of background noise, like restaurants and public spaces. The directional microphone allows the user to focus on the sound source they wish to listen to, and to reduce amplification of conversations behind and to the sides. It is common for such a hearing aid to have both a directional microphone and conventional microphone. Thus user can switch between them as the situation warrants.

Modern digital signal processing has allowed hearing aid designers to develop devices that can actively reduce background noise. These require a fairly significant level of processing, and techniques are continuously being developed in order to increase the effectiveness of the hearing aid. While it is desirable to increase the signal to noise ratio, it is often hard to discriminate the desired sound from the background noise.

Digitally programmable hearing aids can be programmed to have a variable frequency response. They can also be setup to have a series of different settings that are appropriate for different situations and levels of background noise. The user can switch between the different settings as needed.

While telecoils have been available for some time, more hearing aids are being developed with a direct audio input, or DAI. This allows the hearing aid to be connected to an external audio source like a CD player or television. This is preferred by many over a telecoil, as there is less interference. DAI is usually available only in behind the ear hearing aids. They usually use a wire to connect the hearing aid to the external source.

Recent advances in hearing aid technology include the use of wireless technology. This would have the same purpose as direct audio input, without the wires. A person with a wireless hearing aid would also have an FM transmitter that they could hook up to the television, or to a clip on microphone that could be given to someone they wish to have a conversation with.

Disposable Hearing Aids

Disposable hearing aids are simpler than conventional hearing aids. They are currently being marketed to the baby boomer population, with the thought that devices that can be cheaper for people with only mild or moderate hearing loss. Unlike conventional hearing aids, they are not custom-fitted. They usually cannot be adjusted, and instead come in a variety of configurations or prescriptions, selected to match the user's level of hearing loss. A disposable hearing aid's batteries cannot be replaced. They are designed to be thrown out after the batteries expire, which usually last for just over a month. Disposable hearing aids will offer similar quality as a conventional analog hearing aid.

The idea behind disposable hearing aids is that they will appeal to those people who are not sure if they need a hearing aid, and do not wish to spend the money required to purchase a conventional hearing aid. Disposable hearing aids usually cost between $40 and $50 each. This compares to a conventional digital hearing aid which can cost up to five thousand dollars for a pair. While a conventional hearing aid should last for about five years, the overall price of disposable hearing aid may be slightly more expensive. However, there is not as much money tied up in the device at any one time, making replacement much easier. A disposable hearing aid can be available immediately after a hearing test. There is no need to wait for it to be manufactured like a conventional hearing aid. The potential cost of repair or replacement batteries is eliminated as if the device breaks; you just throw it out and get a new one. If the device is lost or dropped, the cost of a replacement is far less than for a conventional hearing aid.

While disposable hearing aids are sometimes described as one size fits all, they actually fit about 80% of adult male ears and about 60% of adult female ears, although some products advertise a higher rate of match. Most disposable aids are of the in the ear type. However, instead of being molded to the ear, they make use of a soft cap that provides an acoustic seal about halfway down the ear canal.

A disposable hearing aid does have a short life span. They cannot be custom fit, meaning they may be uncomfortable for some people. And disposable hearing aids are not as flexible as modern digital hearing aids, which can be programmed to respond differently in a wide variety of situations. Perhaps the biggest concern of audiologists about disposable hearing aids is that users of them will not have their hearing checked on a regular basis, leading to potential uncorrected problems.

All About Open Fit Hearing Aids

The number of choices offered for a hearing aid, in the market, is overwhelming. This article talks about open fit hearing aids that are in the market. In the case of an open fit hearing aid, one does not have to wait for the ear mould to be prepared, and then returned to you, this makes the time taken comparatively lesser than the latter. These make your job easier when you get it from the dealer. The open type hearing aids have evolved a lot and are less bulky now, and they even come in various colors, and also in user friendly designs. The quality has also increased, and people are happy wearing the ones that are coming now.

Many people do not accept the point that they require help to function properly. It is not a shame to accept the fact that they need help in hearing properly, but often, people consider this to be a matter of pride, and stay away from hearing aid. The children fear about being teased by others, and also care about the insults that they will have to face from the society to be wearing a hearing aid at this age, and they also feel that the hearing aid diminishes their looks. The adults see it as a sign of getting older.

The open fit hearing aids are referred to as over-the-ear hearing aids, or OTE. These are to make the wearer feel comfortable, as they are fitted behind the ear, and with an invisible plastic tube that goes into the ear near the ear canal.

OTE hearing aids are best for hearing defects of high frequency. You must be knowing that the hearing defects varies from person to person. The loss occurs at different levels, and also at different stages. In case of the open fitting hearing aids, the power given is mainly for the defect due to high frequencies.

There is another name for these OTE aids, they are also referred to as BTE hearing aids, behind-the-ear hearing aids. The tubing is of plastic, the tubing, and the ear mould conduct sound keeping the ear mould open. Open fit aids are best suited for children, but adults also wear them. These usually come in bright colors to attract the kids.

One of the most baffling problems with this device is that the plastic tubing might get cracked. So, one needs to take care of the hearing aid in such a way that it remains protected, both from you and others. You need to take utmost care in protecting this device, as the dear pet of yours might end up chewing the device into pieces.

It is always suggested by experts that one must have his hearing capacity checked before he goes in for a hearing aid. This is because ear is a very complex part in human body, and only a trained professional can give you accurate details that might be missed out otherwise. And, finally, your ears are not to be neglected, you cannot be complete without the listening capacity.

BTE Hearing Aids Deals

Buying a the BTE hearing aids from one of the professionals is going to cost you a fortune. Many people who suffer from loss of hearing find it convenient to be ordering the BTE aids by means of email. Many people believe that they are saving quite some amount by doing so, but, are these deals good enough to be struck, or are they just to fool around?

There are many sound amplifying devices that masquerade in the name of HEARING AIDS. These are the ones that merely amplify the surrounding sound and noises, and don't meet the guidelines posted by the FDA. These devices are cheap and they are poor in quality. These so called hearing aids might cost you a mere $6.99 per ear. You sure will end up being cheated.

One will face the consequences when he or she is not consulting a proper ENT doctor when having a problem related to the ear, and they will eventually have problems after using the product that has been ordered by mail for very cheap price with an intention to save up more money on the hearing aids.

The results of one hearing test is required before a seller sells his hearing aid to the concerned person. Even the mailed product, should not be sent to you without a proper test report from the audiologist. The audiologists are not professional doctors who decide on the medical conditions and illness, but they are mere testers. But, they can send an audiogram that is used to alter the hearing aid settings.

Good deals on behind-the-ear hearing aids can be struck on E-Bay. Recently, a reconditioned aid was sold there for a mere $70. It is a Beltone hearing aid, which is supposedly one of the best companies and a original hearing aid costs over $1000, when being purchased new. The 278 BTE, which is from Siemens is also a famous model, and costs around $200. These are good quality deals on the hearing aids, online.

Some of the sellers who sell their hearing aids online deal directly with the professionals. These are generally sold at very low prices when compared to the thousands of dollars that are usually sold for. A hearing aid from Siemens, named Siemens Intuis is offered for $499, and its original cost lies somewhere around $1800. It consists of even microphones that are directional, and auto phone device, which is a technology that reduces the feedback to a great extent. It is a digitalized aid. Another brand with similar configurations, which has a price slab of $2200 is sold for $399 on E-Bay.

There might be a great advantage in buying behind-the-ear hearing aids with the help of email. It is good to explore the possibilities. You always need to remember and find what you want rather than getting stuck with one notion. And the product you buy must be worth the money you pay. And, more than anything, you need to realize that it is worth spending a few hundred dollars than to spend several thousand dollars. If the hearing aids are not what they say they are, then, it sure is a waste of money. So, think and then shell out your money, even if it is a little costly, you need to keep in mind that your hearing power is back in position.

The Importance Of Hearing Aids

Hearing loss can come about from all different reasons such as from birth, illness, or an accident and even through medication. Exposure to constant, loud noises has resulted in piercing the eardrums in some people resulting in a loss of hearing. Hearing loss becomes a physical challenge and in some cases frustrating although in some cases surgery can aid recovery, or using a hearing aid, or with some a combination of the two. Not everyone can expect a complete recovery, so hearing aids have become important within our society.

Children who have hearing difficulties have been abused, teased, misunderstood and often shunned by other children. A parent may have noticed that their child is ignoring them regularly when spoken to or is not learning as well as another child; so should get them tested for their hearing. Today, children's hearing aids are very attractive so they are not such a burden to wear or unappealing.

Your child can overcome many classroom challenges with hearing aids. It can a make a huge world of difference to your child who has the decision to take notice of the teacher or not during a lesson. A child who has difficulty hearing properly will often give up trying after a while, but they do not have to continue to face this problem when there is help available.

There are many jokes about hearing loss, but when faced with the problem it isn't always a laughing matter. One of the biggest challenges a person has to face is usually their family, and not society itself. Other family members are around the person more on a daily basis and may get irritated at having to repeat themselves all the time, or have to position themselves so that the person who has impaired hearing is facing them and can read their lips or interpret their hand signals. It isn't fair on other members of the family if the television or radio has to be turned up louder. With television, some programs now come with subtitles. Movies on DVD also come with subtitles so the whole family can watch without being disturbed by the member who has a hearing loss.

If a person has to wear a hearing aid, situations can get embarrassing if they misunderstand what another person is saying or they laugh at inappropriate moments. Whispering cannot be understood by this person, so a crowd situation needs more careful handling. Some people are insensitive and may make fun of the person who can't hear properly. A person's self esteem can be affected or lowered and can lead to depression from not being able to hear properly, or constantly struggling to understand others or for others to understand their problem. It can be quite a struggle if you feel like an outcast and not able to get the help that you need. Hearing aids will not solve all the problems of a person with a hearing loss, but they do go some way to enriching a person's life by making it easier to communicate.

For a person with a hearing aid, it is quite a struggle trying to use the telephone. There are special aids which can be bought that are equipped with the features needed for phone transmissions, or for using a cell phone.

What Does Siemens Have To Offer?

Siemens which is often misspelled as Seimens, are a business for selling hearing aids. The business has been running for over 100 years (from 1847) with its unusual name and may have suffered for as many years through wrong spelling. The spelling may be confusing, but the hearing aids are not so. Representatives are available and have been trained specially to help you decide what is best suited to your requirements.

The Siemens have a clear understanding how hearing loss has occurred through birth, childhood diseases, an ear infection that couldn't be controlled, through medication or a head injury. People often take loud noises too lightly and not aware of the risks until one day they realize they've lost the ability to hear properly and that they need a hearing aid. Siemens realize the importance of being evaluated essentially so that a person gets the aid and proper fit for them, and when it comes to children they know the importance of caring for their hearing problems.

The Siemens BTE aids benefit children greatly due to their durability. For those who have an active child they know the importance of having something that their child has to use, must be able to withstand the rugged lifestyle they lead. Your child should be given the same chance and any to enjoy life and not miss out due to the limitations hearing aids can impose or not being able to meet their needs.

If you are a frequent traveler with your work, you should ask your Siemens representative about places where you can stop at for service should you require it for your hearing aid. Keep a list for future reference with all your other important paperwork so it is on hand when you need it. The company is very widespread, with locations in Africa, America, Asia, Australia, Europe and the Middle East.

Do you have conductive hearing loss? If you do you should equip yourself with an aid with the primary function that will send sound through the middle or outer ear. Amplified aids will simply restore your hearing, so you will find that analogue aids are ideal for you. Help with your hearing becomes a bit more complicated if it is associated with age or some other cause.

Hearing Aids Inside Out

Whatever type of hearing loss you have, Siemens will have a hearing aid that will improve your life.

Siemens offer a choice in value Digital, Basic Digital, and Ultimate Digital choices. They include the feature of Autophone, which is a big step towards helping a hearing aid user who have been unable to use the telephone properly with their old hearing aid. Among the product families Siemens have the Music Pro, Phoenix Pro, Prisma 2 and the Triano. It is only the Prisma 2 basic BTE model which starts from $1700 upwards.

Siemens participate in educational conferences and in trade shows. They have an event calendar which they can provide you with along with a support program, their marketing and website services. This company is able to help you to purchase a hearing aid, or you may want to sell them, or set up a program in your school or business to raise awareness of hearing loss and hearing aids. They have charity project partners including the Children to Children Project, the Line Of Safety Civic Association and the Pangea Foundation.

Where To Find Discount Digital Hearing Aids

If you are looking around to buy a digital hearing aid, you will want to find a quality aid at the most affordable price. You may have to look a while but you can come across some good discount digital hearing aids.

Your ENT doctor will give you some recommendations on what to buy but not where to get a discount digital hearing aid. Your audiologist isn't likely to know where the best deals are either. The best place to look for hearing aids at an excellent, cheaper cost is by surfing the internet.

Take note that the internet have some sellers who offer discount digital hearing aids which come with an FDA waiver. This comes with the agreement that even if they have sold you the hearing aid, it is down to you to make sure that you have seen a doctor who has ruled out any medical reason which may have caused your particular hearing loss. The seller's waiver is merely to say that you will not hold them responsible for your hearing aid , as it is up to you.

When you have signed the waiver, they can let you to buy a discount digital hearing aid, which do not meet the approval of your doctor. An audiologist will still be needed to give you a hearing test, or audiogram, so that the boundaries of your hearing loss can be defined and any other work to prepare you before you order a hearing aid. Some audiologists work in a clinic without an ENT doctor, so you do not always see a doctor.

There are many hearing aids that come into the very inexpensive category. There is a company that can give you a Build Your Own Digital Hearing Aid at a cost of only $499.50, which is the price of the Ihear digital hearing aid. One seller in digital discount hearing aids is Lloyd's, which have the Rexton Targa2 digital BTE hearing device on offer for only $675. (These are the prices per ear). If someone is not able to buy an expensive pair of hearing aids, these are an ideal starting point even though they are not quite as fancy as the more expensive ones.

You can get discount digital hearing aids which are priced at under $1000 justly so. They come with notable statistics. The Rexton Calibra gives you 4 frequency channels with 3 memories which allow for different settings for various environments. It has a feature which can manage feedback very well. This is an excellent brand of hearing aid as it has sophistication to some level for those people who are not able to afford the ones of a higher brand.

There are some advanced hearing aids which can come with a discounted price at times. The Siemens Acuris CIC comes with programmable e2e technology, with excellent feedback handling, three memory settings for sorting noise and sound then emphasizes sound, and with 16 channels. Siemens price these at $1999, but they are available at $1650 if you look elsewhere.

There are companies which sell many brand name hearing aids at a much reduced value. A discount on hearing aids at 60 percent off the usual price is the claim of Genesis hearing aid labs. You can find another company which promise to give you 50 percent off the price of your hearing aids if you do your own adjustments yourself.

You can find many deals which offer discount on digital hearing aids. Once you have seen a hearing specialist ask them to work out the which aid would suit you the best and which ones they have experience of adjusting. Before you decide to purchase a digital discount hearing aid you need to know what you're looking for.

The Popularity Of Behind The Ear Hearing Aids

For a person who is hearing impaired there are so many choices if they are going to get a hearing device. You can get aids that just go in the ear or ones that fit inside the ear canal completely. One would expect these types to be the most popular for cosmetic reasons. Today the most common of hearing aids to be used are behind the ear hearing aids.

These hearing aids are made up of an ear mould designed to fit in a person's ear which is connected to a piece of tubing onto the hearing aid. The tube is known as the tone hook. The hearing aid will have a control for on and off, a control for volume and the battery compartment. The microphone is situated at the top of the hearing aid. Sound reaches the ear by the tubing, through the ear mould that is in the ear.

In general, children who are fitted with a device for their hearing loss are given behind the ear hearing aids. The reason behind this is that they tend to be much more robust than other kinds. They are easy enough for a child to learn to put an aid in and operate it, with the large controls that they can handle.

Children encounter a few difficulties with behind the ear hearing aids, which are usually minor. As they grow, so will the size of the ear canal and the shape, so they may require a refit twice a year. This can also happen with other styles of hearing aids. A child may have trouble remembering where their behind the ear hearing aid is as it is small when they have removed them, and other types could pose even more problems. With children, some do not have ears that are large enough for a behind the ear hearing aid. They need to be fitted correctly which sometimes helps, but if not a device known as a "Huggy" is available so the aid can be fitted to the head so that it is more secure.

As behind the ear hearing aids are a little larger than other devices which are usually worn in the ear, bigger batteries can be used. This gives more power and increased amplification. For any person that uses a hearing aid, this proves very useful if you have a mild hearing loss to someone who has a more profound hearing loss. If a person has problems with the use of their hands and fingers due to a condition like arthritis behind the ear hearing aids are easier for them to handle with the larger controls. They can have circuitry which is either analogue or the advanced digital technological ones.

Behind the ear hearing aids are powerful, strong and easy to use. For a child they are the ideal choice for many reasons. They come in many styles and colors to give variety. As they now come in digital is it any wonder that they have become very popular as the most used hearing aid today.

Siemens Artis Hearing Aids And Their Popularity

Siemens hearing aids sell very well and on the market they produce 20 percent of the hearing aids on sale. One of their best products is the Siemens Artis hearing aids and there are lots of reasons why they are popular.

The latest model that they have come up with is the Artis 2, with many features that make it more desirable. They are fitted with the e2e wireless technology so that even if you are wearing a hearing aid in each ear this Siemens Artis Hearing Aid acts as one unit. There is no need to adjust one aid to correct the volume then the other as it is synchronized with one button. Each aid is fitted with a microphone to collect sound and the circuitry processes it before sending as sound to the ear. They are different in that they are linked by directionality and control. There is also a remote control device called the ePocket which can control both aids together so that it is easier to work.

The Siemens Artis hearing aids are fitted with a system which collects data about the person and the setting levels and volume that they use the most. Eventually, over a short period the adjustments become automatic, by DataLearning which is like tivo technology. The Artis 2 also has DataLogging, which makes a record of all the data which is useful for the audiologist to read to adjust your aid at the next fitting.

Siemens Artis hearing aids have the advanced technology of being able to distinguish clearly between speech sounds and background noises, so that speech sounds are emphasized. This is done by using the many channels and frequency bands automatically which makes them such a breeze to use.

Siemens Artis hearing aids are also fitted with eWindscreen so that when wind is around your ears and making your hearing aids whistle, it can actually reduce this or cut it out altogether. Feedback is also controlled well, which is the squealing noise you normally hear as someone is putting in their aid or adjusting it. A hearing aid that isn't well made can squeal in other situations but you won't get this feedback at all with a Siemens.

The hearing aids also come with the Autophone feature. This enables a person to be able to talk on the phone whilst they are wearing a hearing aid. When the receiver of the phone is place up to the ear, it automatically comes on, with a small beep to indicate that it is on. It automatically goes off when the phone is taken away from the ear.

Another version of the Siemens Artis hearing aids is the Siemens Artis Life. Most of the features are very much like the Artis 2 - the added bonus is how comfortable it is as a BTE hearing aid and how tiny it is so it is less visible. When a person has to wear ear plugs all day they get the feeling of being clogged up so it is a relief to take them out. This is the occlusion effect which is eliminated with the Artis Life.

This is the best hearing aid on offer by Siemens currently. With its many features which it make it comfortable to wear, with ease of use and its accuracy, it is no wonder the Siemens Artis hearing aid has gained in the popularity stakes.

Why Use Hearing Aids For Dogs?

We all need to hear so we are aware of what is going on around us and expect to be able to use it especially when to alert us of any dangers. Dogs also need to be able to hear, but it is expected that they can adapt to life without it. While some dogs manage, is there any reason why dogs shouldn't use a hearing aid?

Dogs can live up to a good age and easily reach their teens before long. With good veterinary care and modern medicine they can live to a ripe old age. Just like humans, as they get older, they will suffer from conditions that come with age like their hearing.

You will notice when your dog loses its hearing as suddenly he is less responsive when you call his name or may not look up at all. If he is facing you he is more likely to respond. Or when he is called you find that he is looking in the wrong direction. Other signs are that he is sleeping most of the time, and will only wake when you touch him. You may also notice that he is shaking his head around like a child would with hearing problems, and they start to make a fuss of their ears. This is when a hearing aid could come in handy to help your dog overcome these problems.

This is a clinic in Texas which can give a hearing test to any dogs that are brought in with suspected hearing loss. Once the test has been carried out, the dog's owner will have more of an idea of what hearing loss their dog is diagnosed with and if there are any suitable solutions to help them. The centre offers a plans to help dogs get used to wearing a hearing aid. Over a month the volume of the aid is gradually adjusted to the right level for the dog. The price is about $250 for each aid. The programs are designed to ease a dog gently into wearing a hearing aid and get used to the idea with the least discomfort.

There is a contraption available for dogs as a hearing aid which easily fits onto their collar. The aid comes in a container which is collar mounted, with a tube leading from it to a foam plug which is placed in the dog's ear. This is very much structured like the BTE, that is Behind the Ear, hearing aids. These devices tend to be tolerated by smaller dogs, as the larger dogs don't take to them as well.

Hearing Aids Inside Out

There are companies that can offer ITE, In the Ear, hearing aids to suit dogs. A doctor will take a mould of the dog's ear canal, which is then sent on for the laboratory to use and build the human ITE into it. Once that is made the dog has to go through the normal testing before the hearing aid is fitted in his ears, although that could be a difficult step. This is the risk and expense that owners take as some dogs will tolerate a hearing aid and others won't stand for it. Some pet veterinary insurance companies do actually cover the cost of these devices.

A dog is more confident if he can hear his owner's voice. He is also alert to danger around him and can respond when he needs to. Hearing loss can make it confusing for him as he suddenly notices changes in his hearing world. Having a hearing aid will make all the difference and make him happier at coping with life. Any loving dog owner will understand these reasons.

BTE Digital Hearing Aids

Those people that need to use hearing aids find that aids are available to fit on the different parts of or in the ear. There are different types of circuitry in hearing aids. The BTE Digial Hearing Aids uses the latest circuitry with the usual type of hearing device.

It was years before digital processing came about. When it did come out, it was too large and bulky to be practical at all. Once it was possible to use them, they were still impractical and it was only when the technology you get today arrived that circuits became tiny. BTE Digital Hearing Aids uses the advantage of this technology like many other hearing aids.

BTE actually means 'Behind the Ear'. The basic structure of the BTE Digital Hearing Aids are just like the usual BTE aids. There is an ear mould which custom made to fit inside a person's ear. The mould is hooked up to the hearing aid, which just sits behind the ear, using a tube known as the tone hook. The top of the hearing aid has a microphone for channeling sound into the aid. The controls are easy to use on the aid which is both durable and powerful.

BTE Digital Hearing Aids have come a long way from the analogue type that first came out. Try listening to an old vinyl record and compare that to a CD; you hear a distinctive sound difference that digital makes. There is so much more that the aid can do for you.

The function of the BTE Digital Hearing Aids converts the sound picked up from the microphone into computer bits, which are then processed at a surprisingly speedy rate. This is done by a processor called a DSP by the hearing aid industry, which is a digital signal processor.

The DSP works by sorting the sounds into channels of frequencies which are split into lower and higher pitches, that is what speech sounds are made up of. By not getting the full range of these audible frequencies, you will not be able to pick up all the sounds so what you will hear is jumbled up speech. With the BTE Digital Hearing Aids you are given the power to amplify the sound even more so that you distinguish voices much more easier.

These hearing aids treats continuous noise differently to how they process noises which have a shorter duration. For instance, the doorbell ringing would interest you more than the sound of an air conditioner running. Feedback is minimized through the circuitry and the ear mould which fits into the ear.

These hearing aids can also correct the problem of recruitment where a person that has a hearing loss finds that soft noises will sound too soft and also loud noises become too loud. With digital processing of the sound, this is all diminished. Some of these hearing aids come with two microphones so that the wearer can focus on the sound coming from the front, known as directionality. This is to provide less distraction which you can get from the environment surrounding you.

With a BTE Digital Hearing Aids offers the best of both worlds. They are durable enough and so easy that a child can use them, with the added advantage of the modern digital sound processing. It provides better hearing for most.

Choosing Discount Hearing Aids

There are many brands and models of hearing aids today. There are several ways to wear them in or on the ear. When you visit an ENT doctor, or otolaryngologist they will usually make the decision for you if you allow them to. If you want to save money gather some information and take it with when you visit your doctor. You should be able to get discount hearing aids without losing out on quality.

There are sellers who can offer discount hearing aids identical to the ones provided by the manufacturer at full price. The only difference is in the price you pay which can be half price or less than what you would normally be expected to pay. When you find a special deal, be sure that you are getting the same equipment apart from the price.

You should look out for certain features and be familiar about what you are looking for to make sure you are getting the right product for your needs. You also need to check whether you are getting the real product, so that if you are buying a fully digital model it is listed as 100 percent fully or totally digital. You don't want to be landed with a mode that has some analogue components, which will not allow for flexibility and processing that is necessary.

Have a look at the channels or frequency bands. The more channels there are then this is better as the fitter is given more latitude to accommodate your hearing losses through the ranges that are not consistent. Having more channels means that your audiologist can amplify the frequencies and tailor them to your needs so that you get more or less hearing where it is needed. If your discount hearing aid does not have the same channels that you find in the manufacturers' hearing aids, the response to programming will be different.

Look at the data carefully of both hearing aids so that you compare it with the model of the manufacturers as you want to make sure you are getting the same hearing aid with microphones which are the same in directional capability. Not all models have directional microphones so if it is featured in one and not the other, then you are not getting the same as the manufacturer's which is what you were expecting.

You also need to check the memory presets of the hearing aids to see how many there are and the brand name. They will tell you if you are getting what an original brand would offer but at a discount price. We all have personal preferences as more memory is not always better, so just be sure you have an adequate number and type of memory presents that you need.

It is easy to get confused by the number of discount hearing aids available. You can find many BTE hearing aids at lower prices. There are also other types of hearing aids like the ITE, that is 'In the Ear', which fit right inside the ear. Try to recognize the different types of ear canal aids like IC (In the Canal) and CIC (Completely In the Canal).

The final process is deciding on whether you are getting real value for your money. You need to look at the prices of models and styles which claim to be identical to see if you getting a deal that is worthy and reliable. Have a look at the goods policy to see if there is a trial period where you can return the product if you are not happy with it any way. If not it is better to look elsewhere as you don't want to be lumbered with a product you are not happy with. This is the most important factor to consider when you choosing a discount hearing aid.

Good Things To Know About Siemens Hearing Aids

For those who are hearing impaired, Siemens offer many products to choose from in hearing aids. Their most advanced product is the Siemens Centra Active hearing aid. For anyone who leads an active lifestyle there are no limits to what you can do with this kind of hearing aid. This product is also designed to be moisture resistant so if you like to keep fit with sporting activities, or during the summer go for walks, or be out in the garden, you are likely to perspire. Some hearing aid users have experienced problems with their aids from the summer heat or from the menopause which brings on hot flushes. Siemens have nanocoated their hearing aid to repel moisture and prevent corrosion so it makes it more reliable. It means you can enjoy more time outside especially in the Summer without the worry that when you work up a sweat your hearing aid will suddenly go on the blink.

This small instrument also comes with a clip-on microphone cover which it protects it from dust, moisture and even tiny particles like pollen. It can be annoying if you get a build up of pollen during the spring so it is good to have this protection.

Siemens have also come up with the development of the charger so you don't ever have to think about running out of batteries, which can be frustrating for the hearing aid wearer. There is nothing like being caught out without any spare batteries. We already use battery chargers for cell phones, digital cameras and video recorders so now that the technology is available for the hearing impaired is wonderful. Having batteries can be limiting and inconvenient so the Centra Active charger, offers a great help to the hearing aid wearer. Whilst you sleep the smart charger just takes five hours before it automatically switches off once done. You can use your hearing aid for a full day and evening with no worries.

Siemens also offer some other great products:

1 Siemens Acuris Life - $1300, the first wireless aid, an open canal aid with flexible tubes that have soft tips, 16 channels, 3 memory settings and a 3 year warranty

2 Siemens Centra Active - $1600, is rechargeable, water resistant, with an optional charger $150, available in 11 colors

3 SiemensArtis2Life

4 SiemensCieloLife

5 SiemensCielo2Life

6 Siemens Cielo DIR BTE

To determine which hearing aid is best for you tests will be performed on you to measure your degree of hearing loss including: audiometry, auditory brainstem response, emissions, otoacoustic, tuning fork and whispered speech. An audiologist is someone trained to evaluate hearing defects and treat them, and can determine the best type of hearing aid for you by looking at all the data from your tests. With some people there is added bone growth that interferes with how sound waves transmit. Surgery can stop or reverse this problem about 70% of the time. In the meantime, a hearing aid is useful before surgery, or if you still have some degree of hearing loss following surgery it may still be necessary to use one.

Hearing Aids GA: For A Good Fit

The modern hearing aids of today are usually programmed using a computer in one way or another before they are fitted. The technology of Hearing Aids GA was designed to give a fitting that is more precise. An audiologist uses this tool that is relatively new to give you the hearing experience that you desire.

The GA, for Hearing Aids GA, is for genetic algorithms. Firstly, is to look at what algorithms are so as to understand them. An algorithm is determining how something gets done. There are often different ways to do something to achieve a goal. The algorithm is the chosen way of doing something. All algorithms have their advantages and disadvantages, although they all accomplish the same goal basically. We all have varying pathology so we have our own unique algorithm which is used to program a digital hearing aid so that it fits with good results. Each result is different for each user for the fitting of their hearing device.

These algorithms are so called genetic algorithms because the elements found in biological genetic principles are mimicked. One example is natural selection where a set of parameters is discarded if it is found to be weaker or less useful than another set, that is, it does not get selected. Hearing Aids GA does have a few possibilities but is able to do the job of rating each selection and picking out the best one for you.

This will be done when you go for your fitting. The audiologist will normally give you two options as presented by the Hearing Aids GA, and you select the one which you find better. It carries on giving you two options until all the information is processed to arrive at a conclusion according to your preferences.

In one study, subjects with normal hearing were tested by being given speech sounds that were distorted to listen to. The Hearing Aids GA looked at their preferences and programmed to give the overall best solution for the problem, which it did in most cases. A second study was done with the subjects to see if the same preferences came up again in the feedback from a second time. Indeed they were. This technology is proven to give an accurate fitting for the majority of individuals which is excellent.

In order for it to be practical long term and continue to be effective, they should be capable to adjust to a user's change in preferences. Artificial intelligent design is important in these instances in being responsive to the wearer's actual use.

Some Hearing Aids GA now come with Bluetooth technology so that it be downloaded to a program which communicates with the hearing aid. There is where the audiologist comes in as they are the only one professionally trained to do the fitting. They are not developed enough that you can do it by yourself.

It is a great advantage having hearing aids that are digitally programmable. The programming is the most important part and that is what Hearing Aids GA does, so that you get a fitting which doesn't take long and is as accurate as it can be.

How Do Hearing Aids Work?

Hearing aids came about more than two hundred years ago. They first appeared as conical shaped ear trumpets and horns which were held up to the ear so a person could speak into it. Sound travelled down the funnel directly into the hearing impaired person to enable them to hear. Hearing aids have a come a long way since then with many impressive types which work with the higher level of technology today. Now we will look at how hearing aids work in today's modern world.

Hearing aids have small microphones which pick up sound which is then amplified to make it louder. A small microphone receives the sound coming in where it is then converted into an electrical or digital signal, the data is then sent back to a speaker so it becomes sound again. The microphones are set according to a person's hearing loss in their usual environment and will account for that to make hearing as normal as possible. The environment will refer to the usual sound and noises that are around you on a daily basis. If you are around high frequency noises, is it necessary to able to hear them? Are you mainly in an environment where conversation is quiet? The audiologist will ask the relevant questions and then determine how to adjust the settings on your hearing aid to help you. This provides some information for how hearing aids function.

Hearing aids today uses one of the three basic types of technology for converting the signals they receive. The analogue adjustable hearing aid is the cheapest and least advanced. Adjustments are carried out by your audiologist like the volume as well as other specifications. The hearing aid is then custom made to fit you. The volume is controlled automatically, or you can adjust it yourself.

The next type is the analog programmable one which is better than the analogue adjustable as it can be programmed with the use of a computer. The audiologist is able to set the different programs to capture and transmit sound for the differing listening situations that one comes across. As a user you have the option of choosing the program for any given situation, with a remote control.

Hearing Aids Inside Out

The most advanced is the digital programmable hearing aids which work out the more expensive. It took years to perfect the technology as they were impractical or not small enough, and now they are very discreet for the wearer.

So what makes a hearing aid work? The circuitry consists of a feature known as DSP, which is Digital Sound Processing. The utilization of a computer chip takes the sound data and analyses it, then once processed it is then amplified to the ear. The data is made up of billions of digital number codes which are identified and classified into different sounds to give them their correct settings. This data is then converted back into sound which is sent to the ear. As the digital hearing air can identify different frequencies, feedback can be detected and eliminated so there is no background interference for the user. This is what makes it much better than the analogue types, as they work automatically and usually need little or no adjustment.

With advancing technology hearing aids just get better and smaller, offering many options for the hearing impaired. They are barely noticeable which make it less embarrassing to wear one, so if you haven't already, you should go ahead and improve your hearing.

How Low Cost Hearing Aids Can Change Your Life

Only the very few can get insurance to cover the cost of their hearing device. For most people they have to get their own help to cope with hearing loss. For many hearing aids are too expensive because of the ridiculous prices that some manufacturers charge. If they are not able to get any assistance, there seems to be not much hope if they want to improve their hearing. If you belong in this category, there are solutions that could help you. Low Cost Hearing Aids could be just the thing to improve your life.

By logging onto a computer, you can surf the internet for many offers by sellers who sell brand name hearing devices rather than directly from the manufacturers. Often you can save money as these sellers are selling the hearing aids which you want but at an affordable lower cost. As the prices are more competitive you can look to buy a hearing aid that is more advanced technologically and more stylish than you thought possible. You don't have to miss out.

With Low Cost Hearing Aids you can hear voices much more clearly again with no distraction of background noise. With the technology of data learning functions, they can be adapted for your particular style of listening. This is the advantage of being able to buy at low cost so that you can afford these extra features.

If your hearing aids comes with directional microphones, you should be able to hear what is facing you quite clearly. You don't have to worry about any noise that is behind you, as long as the sound that you are trying to hear is in front of you. Some models come with a switch so that if want to hear everything that is around you, the directionality can be turned off.

If you have problems hearing certain frequencies, such as children's voices some of which are high pitched, there are some Low Cost Hearing Aids which are available with several channels. This allows your hearing aids to be adjusted according to your hearing needs with the many channels or frequency bands which can be set to your range. This will be done by your audiologist. As your hearing changes so these settings can be changed again.

Hearing Aids Inside Out

There are people who suffer from a condition called recruitment, where sound can be too quiet one moment and then suddenly sound too loud. There are some Low Cost Hearing Aids which come equipped with a feature to cut down on the problem and also has control over feedback.

There are many hearing aids that come with memory presets. If you have one that is identical to one that a manufacturer has at a higher price, it might have several memories which can cope with the different listening environments.

We all rely on being able to use the telephone on a daily basis, so it is disabling if you're not able to use it. There are devices available on many of the Low Cost Hearing Aids which allow a person to listen to the telephone better. Some can actually work with cell phones which is good if you are out and about.

The Variety Of Oticon Hearing Aids

Any two people will expect different things from the use of a hearing aid. Some have a hearing aid allow them to hear properly again so it is practical to have one for that very reason. There are some who are concerned about the cosmetic aspect and how they will look wearing the device. Many will look at the price before they buy. With Oticon Hearing Aids there are choices to suit everyone.

There are an assortment of models that come in many styles, the technological advancement and types which all come with a range in prices. Each Oticon Hearing Aids will focus on certain aspects of the hearing experience.

The Go Pro is a model that is reasonably inexpensive. This aid provides excellent sound quality in digital features. The device is simple yet complete with automatic features. This selection is good for someone who doesn't want to spend on much or compromise on the quality that comes with Oticon hearing aids.

The Atlas is also a model that is lower in cost. It is more economical as it has been designed to made by robots on an assembly line. This may not be appreciated by some, but it is something to consider when looking at price.

There are different models available at Oticon to cope with all levels of hearing loss. Generally all the hearing aids are for mild to moderate hearing loss. If you have a very mild hearing loss there is the Delta model designed just for this. If you have severe hearing loss you will find the best choice is the Sumo DM. It is possible for the wearer to hear voices more clearly and strongly with less distortion. Batteries also last longer than some high power aids which consume power quickly.

The Safran focuses on different aspects that is found on most; the user is able to hear other sounds rather than just speech. They can enjoy the world around them much better by listening to the sounds of nature, with more emphasis given to the sounds of speech.

Hearing Aids Inside Out

Oticon have gone one step further to produce hearing aids which are higher technologically and more sophisticated. The Synchro model is made using artificial intelligence that focuses on speech and filters out noise. It can automatically distinguish between noise and sound, filtering out the unwanted noise and emphasizing sound that we want to hear.

Oticon also offer the Epoch hearing aid so the wearer is able to distinguish easier where sound is coming from and can be used with mobile phones. The Rise is a model which has Bluetooth enabled technology and can also be used with MP3 players. Oticon have many hearing aids which work with binaural sound, where two hearing aids work together centrally as one processor.

Oticon have come up with the Tego hearing aid which has OpenEarAcoustics which prevents occlusion, when there is the feeling that the ear is being shut off by the hearing aid blocking the ear canal. It automatically changes the aid to suit the changes in the environment.

If it is the first time that you are looking for a hearing aid or you need a replacement, it is good to have a few choices. With Oticon Hearing Aids there is such a variety in the styles and types to choose from each model, with different features that you can have.

Choices In BTE Hearing Aids

When it comes to the excellent choice in hearing aids today they can worn in different styles like BTE (Behind The Ear), ITE (In The Ear), MC (Mini Canal) and CIC (Completely In The Canal). The most commonly used is the BTE Hearing Aids so some manufacturers design special models for those people in mind.

The Sumo DM model is offered by Oticon which is powerful enough for those who have greater hearing loss so that sound is amplified. This increased ability of being able to amplify sound means that voices no longer sound distorted or weak even. Battery life is also conserved in the design, and once the batteries begin to wear down, the performance of the Sumo DM is not compromised. This makes it very practical for the wearer of a BTE hearing aid who has significant hearing loss.

The Widex Senso BTE hearing aid is a high-tech model which comes with lots of fancy features. It if fully digital and processes sound at an exceptional rate, faster than many digital models which cannot. It uses three bands to process sound. The signal is analyzed, regulated for each frequency, then processed before being sent back through the speakers.

BTE Hearing aids can separate speech from noise so that speech sounds on emphasized. The system is also sophisticated enough to eliminate recruitment. Many people that have a hearing loss love this great feature because they usually can't hear a person speak at first, and when they do repeat it in a louder voice, it's like they are being shouted out.

These hearing aids can also deal with feedback as they have directional microphones on each hearing aid. Noises that are constant in the background are reduced, like the sound you get from a refrigerator. There are also special models available for those people that have a more profound hearing loss.

Several manufacturers make the open ear BTE aid, which are comfortable to wear and very lightweight which is very practical. You can even get the ear mould in a variety of designer colors. The ear hooks that an aid is equipped with is made of extremely thin tubing which is quite a bonus. Some of the aid compartments which is the part that sits behind the ear are very small and so light that they are barely noticeable. There is the Siemens Prisma BTE hearing aids which only weighs two grams, although it has two microphones with a couple of memories with a button so you can switch between the two. There is also the Starkey Aries BTE hearing aids which are very small.

The added bonus that you get with open ear hearing aids is that they do not block your ears. A lot of people find that the usual hearing aids shut off their ears which they find very uncomfortable, also you get the extra build up of ear wax. The open air hearing aid does not have this problem as the ear is allowed to breathe, as we say. Many of them also have a special nanocoating which is a substance that covers the aid and repels foreign matter like dirt, sweat and water which can stop the aid working for a while.

Each type of hearing aid offers advantages for one user or another. When you look at BTE hearing aids, you should examine the options that are on offer carefully before you decide on the best solution for you. For each category you will find many choices.

The Importance Of Getting The Best Hearing Aid

As a young child do you remember the game you used to play with a friend with two paper or plastic cups which were connected with a length of string, so that you each held one and used it like a telephone. This was passed down through many generations as a hearing experiment for a pretend telephone. It became an inspiration for the earliest type of hearing aid - this device was known as the ear trumpet. It was a helpful device for the hard of hearing, but doesn't come close to the hearing aids we get today. The improved development through the years has really come on since the old days.

Hearing is the process of being able to perceive sounds, and 'Otosclerosis' is the medical term for hearing loss.

Getting the best hearing aid will help you overcome the barriers that you have to face every day which other people don't understand is a challenge for you. You will find your communication improves as you can better understand what is going on around you. It isn't easy being made fun of if you can't hear a person or interpret what is being said to you straightaway. For a child it can be quite devastating, as it is a challenge trying to overcome the physical handicap. Once a child receives a hearing aid they are given more courage and their stress is eased a lot.

For many who have a hearing loss the importance of sign language and lip reading can be very helpful, although these tools are not learned by every person who is hearing impaired. They are not helpful in every situation.

Once you realize that you need the help of a hearing aid, there are many things to think about. Think of how much hearing loss you have suffered and whether it affects one or both ears, and how much loss there is in each ear. You will need to look for a hearing aid provider and decide on what is best for your particular ear shape; how much it will all cost for the equipment and batteries. What aid would best suit your lifestyle and what testing you need to decide on your needs. If you have a child with a hearing loss, this is usually picked up by the school nurse when they are given hearing tests. Apart from this you will want to give your child the best, with the options that are widely available in designer hearing aids that come with a choice of colors.

Hearing Aids Inside Out

Having an attractive aid will help your child progress as they are encouraged and take more interest in wearing a hearing aid.

There are many top hearing companies on the market such as Beltone, Phonak, Rexton, Sebotek, Siemens, Sonic Inovations, Starkey, Unitron and Widex. The 'Miracle Ear' is popular and attracts the attention of everyone as there are ads everywhere in magazines to interest the elderly, there are flyers in doctor's practices and many other places. When we think of hearing aids, we think of the elderly, but it is surprising just who wears one nowadays! It isn't just the elderly who get a hearing loss, as this can be developed at any age. If you know someone who wears a hearing aid, you can ask them what their experience is like wearing one to give you some ideas on what you should choose.

Looking at hearing aids, you will find the best ones come with added extras such as an ear wax cleaning tool, instructions, a storage case, spare batteries, a good warranty and phone numbers of service centers to call if you experience a problem or have some questions.

Beltone Hearing Aids

The outside ear is only to receive and concentrate the sound waves, which vibrate in air inside the auditory canal. The air is the one that passes it on to the eardrum. Hammer bone, which is located inside is connected to the stirrup and anvil bones, which is vibrated by the round window and the oval window. This transports the fluid over to the cochlea, where the Organ of Corti is enclosed. This organ is covered up with numerous hair cells, which are tiny, and manage to bring about a chemical change that changes the electrical potential to bring about nerve impulses. The little ear that is by the side of the head is the starting of this process called hearing. It is a very complex method. This is not it, there is a lot more, and the Beltone Company are experts at this.

The Beltone hearing aids are in business for the past 68 years, since 1940. They have a wide range of varieties in hearing aids. The best ones are, Beltone Linq, Beltone Edge, Beltone Arca, Beltone Corus, Beltone Access, Beltone Mira, Petite, Opera Plus, and the Invisa.

The Beltone Hearing Aids have helped numerous generations, and have never let down individuals, and families that relied on their business. They also provide other needs apart from hearing aids, they include amplified cordless phones, Bluetooth ear sets priced at $145, Loud Alarm Clocks, Neck loops priced at $150, personal listening systems priced at $200, and phone modules priced at $50.

The listening system from Beltones help you hear things comfortably in theatres also. Generally, it is hard for a person to hear things in a noisy place, even if he is not hearing challenged. Many people have missed out a lot when they were reading lips in theatres, concerts etc. They have not got the full satisfaction that any other normal person gets after being to one such place. This given situation can be very annoying.

The hearing impaired persons had a problem waking up early in the morning, even when they were equipped with hearing aids. Many people remove their aids when they go to sleep, but when they find the need to be doing so, they realized how uncomfortable it is, to sleep with them. Generally, a timer is put on a light, and when the light is switched on, they wake up because of the brightness. But, this is of no help to people who can sleep, no matter what happens. But, timers cannot be the savior when we are out on trips, and wake up calls and knocking the door cannot wake them up, because they cannot hear. But, nowadays, people don't see the need to worry, because Beltone has come up with their new vibrating wake and shake alarm which is sold at a mere $70. This is incorporated with a vibrating facility, which is activated at the time the alarm has been set.

Beltone is serving people across Canada, New England, and the whole of United States.

Apart from this, even batteries are sold by them. They are available even in many small shops. The pharmacies have batteries for the hearing aids. A good branded battery is sold at a price of $6, for which we get 4 batteries. The batteries can be ordered from AARP magazines. Usually, bigger bundles are sold in such a case, say, you will get 42 batteries for $25. And, your money is refunded, in case you are not satisfied.

Phonak Hearing Aids

It is not possible to pay attention to what is around you all the time. It is even harder for people who have troubles in hearing. The sounds produced seem so muffled, and like they are coming from far away. The voices, somehow, cannot be deciphered. And, some of the hearing aids do nothing but amplifying sound, so, even the unwanted noise is amplified. The Phonak hearing aids here, is meant to make listening a easier process for people suffering from hearing defects.

These hearing aids come at a different level of technology. The least advanced ones are the Analog. These hearing aids are manually changed, and they do not adjust themselves to an individual's preference in an automatic way. All the do is, receive the sound and amplify them.

There are hearing aids that are digitally programmable, and they can be programmed using the computer software. This is one of the greatest advantage of the digital Phonak listening aid. They have settings that are pre-programmed.

Digital Phonak hearing aids really shines. It has a good digital technology backing it up, and is the best suited for your personal preferences. This begins with fitting, but does not end right there.

As you start using the Phonak hearing aids, you will naturally be able to set the volume according to the way the noise around you is. You will adjust automatically, depending on the surrounding, like a crowded football arena, or the quiet atmosphere in a monastery. After sometime, the self learning process involved will make you adapt yourself according to the given situation, and you will adjust your volume accordingly.

There is an option to self log in your Phonak hearing aids, which stores the information about your choice of the volume for a particular situation, that is given by the audiologist. Then, there is a feature called the Auto Pilot, where the hearing aid will automatically set its volume depending on the preset adjustments. The Surround Zoom is another feature that diminishes the noise from the surrounding.

The Phonak Hearing aids also offer one type of aid called the Micro Power, which is tiny. It is powerful enough to help people with acute hearing losses. It is a BTE hearing aid. It's speaker rests on the back of the ear. The tubing that is given for this hearing aid is very small. All the Micro Style hearing aids are small in size, both in the case of tubing and the hearing aids. They are feather light.

These hearing aids come in usual styles. These are ITE hearing aids, called In-the-Ear Hearing aids. ITE hearing aids are fine if the hearing defect is not all that bad. The BTE hearing aids, or Behind-the-Ear hearing aids are accurate for the user with any level of hearing defect, and also for the children.

No hearing aid is capable of giving back what you have lost, your capability to hear without any aid. But, it can be corrected, and with the best, in the form of Phonak Hearing Aids. This makes hearing simpler for you.

Siemens Artis Hearing Aids May Be The Solution For You

There are a gazillion options to choose when you go down to the market to purchase a hearing aid. Siemens tops the list when it comes to manufacturing this device, with an idea to make listening easy for the hearing impaired individuals. A professional will be able to give you a perfect picture as to what you will need.

There is a term called 'Occlusion' when you are referring to hearing aids. This is about something that blocks the passage. Some hearing aids you fit, might make you feel like you are having a cotton ball stubbed up your hear. This occlusion might make you feel bad that you are a hearing impaired person. Occlusion can be best explained when you try listening to someone who is standing above water and talking to you when you are actually under water. You don't need to feel intimidated with the technical terms used when one is discussing about the hearing defects. The one who helps you with the problem will surely able to explain to you the complexities involved.

Siemens offers hearing aids that have a digital noise management technology, and speech enhancement, and also a feedback management; it also includes wind noise reduction. There are four types of Artis hearing aids - the BTE, the ITC, the ITE and CIC. All these cost about $1600.

Hearing Aids are not just meant to help you hear; it should be able to filter the noise and increase the clarity and control the loudness. If your ear sustained damages due to unhealthy exposures, then, one needs to stay away from loud noise in order to prevent further damage. Both the aids must function in tandem. The ones that Siemens make compliment each other and work as a pair. The Siemens Artis e2e hearing aids are available at $1500. With this hearing aid, you do have control to the adjustments manually, but they work in a synchronized manner. The remote further enhances your control over the hearing aids. It works with either one aid, or with a hearing aid in both the ears.

Siemens Artis 2, is a hearing aid that is available for $1100. The feedback in this aid is prevented, thus, it does not give any sort of a squealing sound. A high pitch squealing sound can scare the person if it is going to happen once too often. This hearing aid has the capability to adapt itself, and it has a microphone that can make you get the most out of this system. It also adjusts itself for telephonic conversations, and it has a battery that lasts for 120hrs.

Siemens Artis S has remote control that has volume controls in that, and this aid is used by people with moderate hearing hassles.

The Artis hearing aid offered by the Siemens company is also available as full shell, canal, half shell, mini canal, and also CIC, and its price varies from $1350 - $1450. They are also available with remote controls that are available for $150.

Starkey Hearing Aids

The hearing aids have technically advanced a lot, they are so well advanced that they even let the user listen to iPods! The telephone amplifiers that are inbuilt can be carried along with you to trips. There are even devices that the hearing impaired can take to the theatres which helps them to watch movies without any problem, and it even reduces the noises in the background.

The Starkey is one of the most popular company that is on the top of the list for innovations related to these products. They are making hearing aids that appeal even to the kids of the present generation. If your kid has a problem using the hearing aid, then, his feelings need to be respected, because it is a question of pride. The Starkey company sure will be able to help them with this. They care enough to help the children who are facing hearing impairments.

It would be of great help if the kid first tries the hearing aids on at home for a short duration before it starts using it in school. They will have to get used to the feeling of wearing an aid, and they might need some help to erase the feeling that they are inferior to the others in school. They will have to be taught how to handle the hearing aids in such a way that they do not get damaged. It is good to find other kids who are also wearing hearing aids, and let your child communicate with such kids, it will be of great help. There are many other places that will help your kid eliminate the inferiority complex.

Starkey Hearing Foundation provides aids to many people who have the necessity to be using one. This establishment is located in Minnesota. The Starkey has come up with a program called Star Kids, that will help both the kids and their parents learn about the hearing aids and their functions. You might be needing one for yourself, and you might want to help your child understand the complexities of this better.

Starkey Laboratories uses was a small ear mould company that was later stabilized as a hearing device company by W.F. Austin who merged his company with the existing company. Now, this establishment is spread over 24 countries.

The Starkey aids also come with various features that have a diagnostic tool that will give you proper performance report. It will also remind you about the next visit. In case you are looking for the best, Destiny 1600 is the best, that costs about $2400. The best ones will cost a lot, but are worth it, because the have distinct features. If basics are enough, then, Starkey has no problem in giving them to you.

There are other models:

Davinci PSP line: $2200
Starkey A13 Sequel MMP BTE-1
Sierra line: $1700
Aspect Xtra: $2100
Starkey's Axent line: $2100
Starkey A13 MPT-1

These models are pretty famous in the market, and are preferred by most people, and they are suggested by professionals.

Elton John, Ronald Reagan and Jay Leno are famous people associated with Starkey.

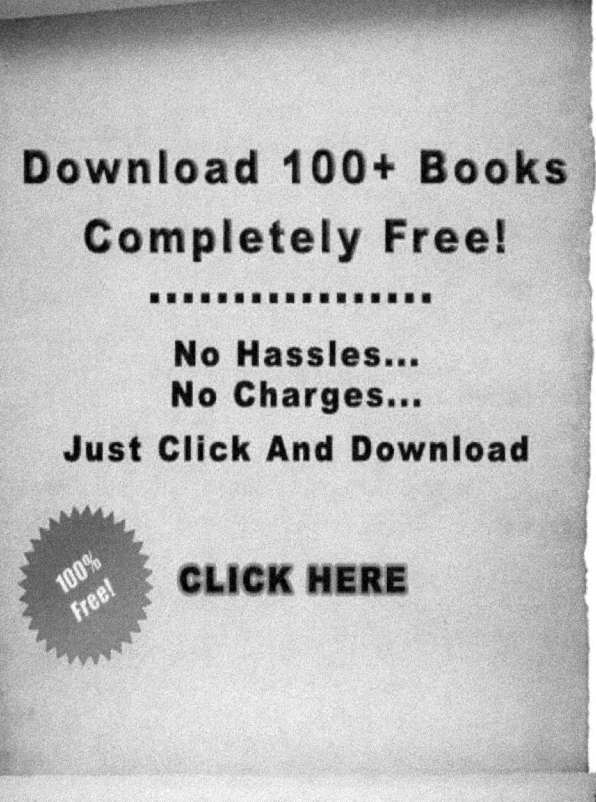

This Product Is Brought To You By

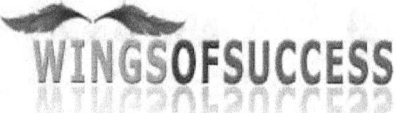

www.ingramcontent.com/pod-product-compliance
Lightning Source LLC
LaVergne TN
LVHW012120070526
838202LV00056B/5809